DEAR LIFE

RACHEL CLARKE

DEAR LIFE

A Doctor's Story of Love and Loss

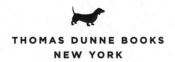

THOMAS DUNNE BOOKS
NEW YORK

Library of Congress Cataloging-in-Publication Data

Names: Clarke, Rachel (Physician), author.
Title: Dear life : a doctor's story of love and loss / Rachel Clarke.
Description: First US edition. | New York : Thomas Dunne Books, 2020. |
  Originally published: London : Little, Brown, 2020. |
Identifiers: LCCN 2020016411 | ISBN 9781250764515 (hardcover) |
  ISBN 9781250764522 (ebook)
Subjects: LCSH: Clarke, Rachel (Physician) | Physicians—England—Biography. |
  Terminal care. | Hospice care. | Palliative treatment.
Classification: LCC R489.C54 A3 2020 | DDC 610.92 [B]—dc23
LC record available at https://lccn.loc.gov/2020016411

To Dave, Finn and Abbey, with love

Contents

Author's Note

The stories told here are grounded in my clinical experience, but elements have been changed in order to protect the confidentiality of staff and patients. In addition, details of the situations and the people I have met and cared for have, at times, been merged or altered in order to further protect privacy and confidentiality. I am extremely grateful to Dr Helgi Johannsson; Andy Taylor; Alice, Sharon and Jonathan Byron; and Diane and Ed Finch for allowing me to tell their stories using their real names.

Tell me, what is it you plan to do
With your one wild and precious life?

Mary Oliver, 'The Summer Day'
from *House of Light*

DEAR LIFE

Prologue

There isn't enough of anything
as long as we live. But at intervals
a sweetness appears and, given a chance,
prevails.

Raymond Carver, 'The Author of Her
Misfortune', *Ultramarine: Poems*

Two men enter an empty studio. They sit down and talk at length over a bottle of white wine, finally departing before drugs lay claim to the eloquence of one of them. Wreathed in smoke, a cigarette permanently clenched in one arthritic hand, the acclaimed British screenwriter and dramatist Dennis Potter has been told the month before that he is dying. The hip flask he sets down on the table beside the wine contains not whisky but morphine. As his interview with the arts broadcaster Melvyn Bragg unfolds, Potter will need televised swigs from the flask to blank out the pain of his inoperable pancreatic cancer.

This is 1994. Back then, in Britain, no one spoke in public about terminal cancer, let alone broadcast its assault on their body on prime-time television. But Potter has always loved to shock his audiences into thought, using drama to confront the truths that most disturb us. This evening, he has chosen to dramatise his own, real-time, corporeal decline.

At age twenty-two, a student who happened to be home from her studies, I was tempted to skirt the televised death talk, but my father told me if I did, I would regret it. And so we sat side by side, in front of the television, as I tried to disguise my discomfort at Potter's dependence on his opiates – this unadorned proximity to dying. Since Dad, a doctor, did not approve of squeamishness, I kept my unease under wraps.

We were watching, it turned out, Potter's last public words. Two months later, he was dead. Yet he filled the studio, and the minds of those who watched, with the sheer theatricality not of dying but of living. Death's imminence, its claim on his future, had given Potter licence to live like a child in the present. Every second sang.

'The only thing you know for sure is the present tense, and that nowness becomes so vivid that, almost in a perverse sort of way, I'm almost serene,' he said, the paradox prompting a lopsided grin. 'You know, I can celebrate life . . . Last week looking at [the blossom] through the window when I'm writing, I see it is the whitest, frothiest, blossomest blossom that there ever could be, and I can see it. Things are both more trivial than they ever were, and more important than they ever were, and the difference between the trivial and the important doesn't seem to matter. But the nowness of everything is absolutely wondrous.'

For a moment – and I knew it was the same for Dad – I felt like I had been handed the key to everlasting happiness. Experience the world with the heightened intensity of a child.

Inhabit now, not tomorrow, or a sad trail of yesterdays. Seize it. Live the moment like it is your last. Needless to say, the humdrum anxieties of everyday existence soon blotted any nowness from my mind. As Potter himself put it so beautifully: 'We're the one animal that knows that we're going to die, and yet we carry on paying our mortgages, doing our jobs, moving about, behaving as though there's eternity.'

In 2017, twenty-three years after Dennis Potter died, his words were resurrected in my mind. Dad, my dearest Dad, was now himself a dying man. In thrall to a cancer not of the pancreas but the bowel, he had spent half a year on the chemotherapy carousel. Infusions, blood tests, nausea, fatigue, infusions, damaged nerves, infusions, bleeding skin. Hope, more than anything, kept him coming back for more. Even when the scans showed terminal spread, still he yearned, burned, for more life. He took them, these monthly batterings of the cytotoxic drugs, because they gave him a space in which to believe. They allowed him to imagine a future.

We all, including Dad, feared his days were running out. Unable to stop time, we groped for moments of timelessness. If we could help him, I reasoned, inhabit the blossom, then perhaps he could elude the doctor's curse – too intimate a knowledge of how his days would likely end, as cancer picked off organs one by one.

I thought back to the tales he had always loved to share of life as a young medic in swinging sixties London, all vibrancy, colour and chaos. Partying hard until the early hours, then driving his scarlet MG sports car through the deserted East End because, in those days, no one cared about drink driving. Skedaddling at dawn from his hospital to the pub around the corner to share early-morning pints with the meat men from Smithfield Market, in boozy, bloodied celebration of surviving three whole days and nights on-call. And, every summer, queuing for cheap tickets to that music festival of world renown the BBC Proms, where he would stand high in the canopy of the Royal Albert Hall as Tchaikovsky and Mahler transported him yet higher.

Music, I was certain, was for Dad a form of blossom. In 'Trenchtown Rock', Bob Marley sang of its power: 'One good thing about music, when it hits you, you feel no pain.' And so, that spring, I secretly booked us seats inside the Albert Hall for an early Prom in the summer of 2017. Berlin's Staatskapelle orchestra would be playing one of Dad's favourite pieces, Elgar's Second Symphony, conducted by the great Daniel Barenboim. Whether Dad would be alive then, or fit for trips to London, I could not say. I suppose the tickets were a talisman, tucked deep inside a bedside drawer, my own small leap of faith into the future.

For Britons, 2017 often felt like the year of hate. Acts of terror came like rain. First, in March, a British-born terrorist, Khalid Masood, ploughed his car through pedestrians on London's Westminster Bridge, killing four of them, before stabbing to death a police officer guarding the entrance to Parliament. Two months later, another terrorist, Salman Abedi, exploded a bomb in the foyer of the Manchester Arena, killing twenty-two concert-goers, including children. In June, another eight people were murdered when terrorists drove a van into pedestrians on London Bridge, then embarked on a stabbing rampage in nearby Borough Market.

The country reeled from onslaught to onslaught. Already

bruised from the preceding year's referendum – Britain's decision to leave the European Union had unleashed much division and anger – now we were battered by terror. It was hard to find reasons for hope. Amid the disbelief and rage, the murderous death toll ever rising, we scratched around for comfort where we could. For Dad, like so many, this lay in the innumerable, instinctive acts of courage that unfurled, like little miracles, from the hate.

'Have you heard about the nurse on London Bridge?' he asked me on the phone one night.

While terrified pedestrians had scattered from the men intent on killing, Kirsty Boden, a twenty-eight-year-old nurse in the NHS, had chosen to run towards the danger. The price of her selflessness, as she stooped to help a victim, was to be fatally stabbed in the chest herself. Her impulse to save others claimed her life.

'If ever one person showed us how much there still is to believe in,' Dad mused, as we asked ourselves whether we, both doctors, would have acted as bravely.

By the time July bathed Britain in sunlight, Dad had been stripped of all his strength by cancer, even as London was reinforced by newly sprouted concrete barriers, placed wherever large groups of people congregated, enticing the men with their vehicles, guns and blades. I had not dared hope for midsummer. But Dad, though frail, was still with us. Overjoyed, I drove my parents to the parking place, booked months earlier, right beside the Albert Hall, in case he was too weak to walk.

Slowly, arm in arm, we climbed the steps towards the hall. Dad's bones were sharp against my skin. The slabs of anti-terror concrete perturbed us. 'Has it really come to this?' he asked. 'That going out to hear a symphony could be life-threatening?'

He bought Mum and me a pre-concert glass of champagne. I had worried he might try to hide his fatigue, feigning enjoyment for our benefit, while really feeling too spent for pleasure. But, as he sipped his drink, the eyes that roved across the crowds glinted bright as bubbles. My heart lurched. It was just as I had hoped.

We took our seats. 'Well,' he grinned, easing his gaunt frame into velvet-covered plushness, 'this isn't quite what I remember from standing up in the roof in the 1960s.' In choosing our seats, I had blown the budget on cancer-friendly opulence. We sat in a box, no less, looking down upon the stage. Beneath the cavernous domed ceiling, the tiers of gilded seats and stage lights, Dad no longer looked frail, but radiant. A hush, reverential, descended. The orchestra entered and, at Barenboim's signal, Elgar's opening notes swelled inside and around us.

I forgot the voice that had dogged me for months, asking, on every visit to my parents, 'How many more times are there left to see Dad now?' I forgot how much it hurts to love someone while losing them. I stole a glance at Mum and Dad, to see him squeeze her hand and smile. Bob Marley was right. Music, if fleetingly, had just cured cancer.

As the orchestra rose to rapturous applause, I knew I would seal this memory away in the back of my mind where it too, in time, might become talismanic. But the blossom, remarkably, was yet to come.

Barenboim turned from the stage to his audience and, breaking with convention, began to address us directly. Though he insisted his words were not political, 'but rather of a human concern', they were sufficiently newsworthy to fill the next day's press, incurring social media wrath and outrage. Speaking as an Argentinian-born Palestinian citizen who had once lived in Britain, and now in Germany, he spoke of his fears of isolationism and – to deafening applause – of music's unique ability to transcend national boundaries: 'If a French citizen wants to learn Goethe, he must have a translation. But he doesn't need a translation for the Beethoven symphonies. This is important. This is why music is so important.'

To some, his words signified an unwanted rebuke of those Britons who had voted, in the previous year's referendum, to leave the European Union. But his appeal for more education 'about who we are, about what is a human being, and how is he to relate to others of the same kind' seemed to me to deliver an altogether different message. Unity, not division, was Barenboim's aspiration. Music, fundamentally, was his means of connection, of bringing people together, irrespective of difference. 'Our profession, the musical profession, is the only one that is not national. No German musician will tell you, "I am a German musician and I will only play Brahms, Schumann and Beethoven."'

I looked across at Dad and smiled. We had argued so often, with such vehemence, about Britain's role in Europe – he a 'Brexiter' who longed for British sovereignty, me a Europhile who carried her EU passport with pride. Barenboim's words touched each of us deeply, surely proving, with eloquence, his point. Poignantly, within this concert hall newly barricaded inside concrete, he continued, 'Religious fanaticism cannot be fought with arms alone. The real evil of the world can only be fought with a humanism that keeps us all together. Including you. And I'm going to show you I really mean it.'

He turned back towards the orchestra and raised his baton.

Silence. And then, gifted to the hall, two encores. First, 'Nimrod', from Elgar's *Enigma Variations*, my father's favourite piece of music. Then, the most overtly patriotic of all of Elgar's works, his first *Pomp and Circumstance March*, widely known as 'Land of Hope and Glory'. Two profoundly political pieces, steeped in anachronistic overtones of greatness and empire, yet played lovingly, in London, by Berlin's finest musicians. There it was. In music more powerful than any words, in a country beset by division and fear, we were reminded of what we shared.

I could think of none of this, however, as the strings ebbed and flowed. My heart had unravelled at the thought, *'Nimrod', Dad's been given 'Nimrod'*. He loved the piece more than any other, passed on that love to me while I was still a child. Too young to understand words like 'patriotism' and 'empire', I simply observed, as he turned up the volume, the music sweep him upwards, somewhere high. And I felt the brass and drums inside the cave of my chest as thunder, lightning, all the might of the world, somehow distilled into sound. 'Nimrod', I grew up learning, was Dad's anthem, and so, of course, it became mine.

Beneath the auditorium lights, tears shone from my parents' faces as I watched them smile, rapturously. How very unlikely, how outlandish, that now, in using Elgar to plead for our common humanity, Barenboim had unwittingly enabled the dying man in the box right of stage to live, for a moment, wondrously.

In today's developed world it is possible to live an entire lifetime without ever directly setting eyes on death, which, considering half a million Britons and two and a half million Americans will die every year, is remarkable.

Little more than a century ago, this distance from dying was inconceivable. We invariably departed the world as we entered it, among our families, close up and personal, wreathed not in hospital sheets but in the intimacy of our own homes. Now, though, both birth and death have become, by and large, institutionalised. The only two certainties around which our lives pivot have been outsourced to paid professionals. A scant 2 per cent of births in Britain are home births, and only one in five of us will die at home, despite two thirds of us expressing the wish to do so. Hospitals, hospices and care homes are the new repositories of modern-day demise.

Doctors, in involving themselves in matters of dying, therefore do something highly unusual. I am odder than most. By specialising in palliative medicine, I use my training and skills specifically to help people with a terminal illness live what remains of their lives as fully as possible, and to die with dignity and comfort. I have, in short, made dying my day job. Rarely, if ever, does a week go by in which all of my patients survive.

Most people's reaction on learning what I do for a living is to wince as they mutter, 'I don't know how you can bear that.' You can almost feel the suppressed recoil as they shrink from the thought of all that death. And I don't blame them. I used to recoil once too. Losing someone you love can be a pain more searing than any other. And there is no escaping the fact that dying, like childbirth, can be gruelling – though far less commonly than I once imagined. As a patient once told me: 'I'm not afraid of dying, I just never realised it would be such hard work.'

The allure of medicine is easy to understand. There is power, respect, status, gratitude. But why on earth would a doctor, after all those laborious years of study – the hard-won potential to restart a child's heart, give back the gift of sight, reset a shattered limb, transplant a kidney – choose to immerse themselves in death and dying? What could possibly be the attraction of day in, day out grief and sadness, all of it tainted by the whiff of defeat, of inescapable medical failure?

If neurosurgeons are the rock stars of the medical hierarchy – its sexy, alpha, heart-throb heroes – then palliative care doctors are the dowdy support act. A low-rank medical speciality, we lurk in the shadows, too close to death for comfort, murkily intervening with our morphine and midazolam once our charismatic cousins have exhausted their efforts at cure. No one in the hospital is quite sure what we get up to, and usually does not wish to know either. Death is taboo for many reasons, not least the fear that it might just be catching.

Once, shortly after I qualified as a doctor, a consultant oncologist summed up in one sentence a certain old guard's attitude to terminal diagnoses. We had just left the bedside of a patient whose cancer had spread widely, despite her last-ditch chemotherapy. 'There's nothing more for us to do here,' the consultant had said by the sink, as he literally and metaphorically washed his hands of her. 'Send her to the palliative dustbin.'

His words left me dumbstruck. Were there really doctors who dismissed patients as trash, as having lives devoid of value, once medicine could no longer prolong them? At the time I could hardly conceive of a more repugnant sentiment, though today I wonder if the consultant's remark was really a crass attempt at humour, born out of embarrassment and discomfort at his own perceived impotence. The feelings death stirs are nothing if not complicated.

Prologue

Even I – someone who works with death on a daily basis – treat the subject with caution. My own children, for example, still do not know exactly what Mummy does at the hospital, and I am not sure how old they will be before I feel entirely comfortable explaining all. They assume, I imagine, that I save lives for a living. That is, after all, the old medical paradigm. The dramatised doctors who stride across our television screens, swoop in, take command, deploy their skills and save the day. Stethoscopes in place of capes, but doctor-heroes all the same, prolonging life, denying death, playing God with impunity.

When I was a child myself, devoted to my physician father, I came to glimpse through him a different, quieter style of doctoring in which medicine perhaps achieved less yet was kinder and more humane. I learned from his inexhaustible tales that even when a patient's fate seems hopeless, a doctor, if they care, through their basic humanity, can always make things more bearable, and that this was something to emulate. The lesson must have lodged in my brain. Two decades later, upon belatedly qualifying as a doctor myself, I would discover that a frenetic, overstretched hospital environment threatened to stamp out of medicine the very things that had made me most proud of my father – his unassuming attention to his patients, an innate and profound love of people. Exhausted doctors swiftly mutate into burned-out ones who wearily go through the motions of healing.

Perversely, the one part of the hospital that allowed me to flourish as a doctor was the ward most steeped in fear and taboo: the inpatient palliative care unit. If I told you that my work there today is more uplifting, more full of meaning, than any other form of medicine I could imagine practising, you might think too much time in the hospice had addled my brain. But what dominates palliative medicine is not the proximity to death, but the best bits of living. Kindness, courage, love, tenderness – these are the qualities that so often saturate a person's last days. It can be chaotic, messy, almost violent with grief, but I am surrounded at work by human beings at their most remarkable, unable to retreat from the fact and the ache of our impermanence, yet getting on with living and loving all the same.

One way or another, I have circled death and dying for half a lifetime. Like most of us, blithely pretending our days are not numbered, I have had my share of close shaves. Narrowly escaping a terrorist nail bomb, crawling out of the wreckage of a car on black ice, even fleeing bullets from Congolese child soldiers. Then, in choosing to become a doctor, I elected to attend more closely to death – and to the inevitable grief it unleashes. Finally, upon specialising in palliative medicine, I learned that dying, up close, is not what you imagine. For the dying are living, like everyone else. It is the essence of living – beautiful, bittersweet, fragile life – that really matters in a hospice. You would be surprised by what we get up to.

1

Near Misses

We are, all of us, wandering about in a state of oblivion,
borrowing our time, seizing our days, escaping our fates, slipping
through loopholes, unaware of when the axe may fall.

Maggie O'Farrell, *I Am, I Am, I Am*

The first time I remember thinking about dying was as an impressionable seven-year-old. Then, at the height of the Cold War, my early morbid fascination was inspired by Mrs Dewar, my brilliant but idiosyncratic primary school teacher, a woman with the Soviet Union on her mind. Thin and intense, with a piercing stare, she could flip in an instant from subtraction to mutually assured nuclear destruction, holding her young audience rapt and quaking.

'Children!' she would warn us, glowering darkly. 'The Russians are coming. I tell you, the Russians are coming.'

None of us was entirely certain who or what the Russians were, but we were mercilessly brought up to speed. When they came for us, they would slaughter us all, mothers, fathers, brothers, sisters. The world we had happily taken for granted was teetering, all of it, on the edge of oblivion, apocalyptic horrors on the cards at any time. No part of the country, not even the tiny village I inhabited in rural Wiltshire, was impervious to the threat of East–West animosity escalating into full-blown nuclear war. This was too enormous for my young brain to fathom – not a single person's death, but the annihilation of a species, no human being spared. Dread seeped into my bones.

Children are meant to be so absorbed in the vital business of day-to-day living that their own mortality passes them by. But I remember going to bed, aged seven, genuinely fearful I might not be alive in the morning. I would lie awake, rigid with fear beneath the duvet, and when I did sleep, mushroom clouds haunted my dreams. One night, in the small hours of the morning, my father was awakened by the clanking of a clumsy intruder. Stark naked and armed with only a poker, he crept – half superhero, half Benny Hill – into the living room to find not a burglar, gloved and masked, but his sleep-walking daughter, knocking ornaments flying as I groped my way along the window sill, eyes tight shut, muttering my now-internalised dread: 'The Russians are coming, the Russians are coming. We are all. Going. To. Die.' Dad scooped me up in the darkness and tucked me back into bed. I can still recall the feeling of absolute safety, as though nothing could touch me when held in his arms.

My early existential angst at nuclear Armageddon was swiftly superseded by more pressing concerns, like whether seven-year-old Ben Hardy, the boy in my class famed for eating nothing but tomato ketchup sandwiches at lunchtime, would ever agree to marry me. It turned out that, like most children, I was indeed too entranced by living to dwell upon something as abstract and ethereal as dying.

Death, if it cropped up at all, was in the form of illicit entertainment. Every Friday night after school, for example, clean and fresh from our evening baths, my brother, sister and I would eagerly clamber on to the sofa for our weekly treat, on BBC television, of an old black-and-white Tarzan movie. In the title role, Johnny Weissmuller, the Olympic swimmer turned 1930s Hollywood star, ran, leapt and hollered his way through the jungle, his oiled six-pack gleaming. The highlight was never Johnny however, nor even his feral sidekick, a filthy-cheeked child known only as 'Boy'.

What we loved, as only eight- or nine-year-olds can love, was the terrible scene, towards the end of each movie, when a baddie would receive a very special comeuppance. 'It's the tree!' one of us would scream with ghoulish delight, since not all of the movies contained this blood-curdling finale.

'The tree' involved furious natives (as Tarzan referred to them) spread-eagling the baddie upon two crossed tree trunks, then raising him, pinioned, into the sky. His left arm and right leg were tied tightly to one trunk, his right arm and left leg to the other. Far below the hapless baddie, jungle drums beat in a manic crescendo while natives danced themselves into a frenzy. Tarzan himself would be hidden or captured, thus powerless to prevent the imminent slaughter. A machete would be raised, and quiver briefly in the sunshine. Then, all of a sudden, the ropes securing the trees would be cut, a female starlet would avert her eyes in anguish, and the trees would snap apart with a sound like a bullet, ripping the victim clean in half.

'The tree, the tree!' we'd laugh uproariously before descending, every week, into the same heated argument.

'You wouldn't be ripped in half,' one of us would declare.

'Yes, you would! Right down the middle.'

'No, you wouldn't. Your legs would get pulled out of their sockets. And your arms. They'd stay on the tree trunks and your body would fall down and you'd bleed to death.'

'Well, actually, your body would be ripped in half – all the way up to your head – and then your skull would fall off and that's how you'd die.'

And so it went on. Rarely – an extra special treat – Dad arrived home from work in time to perch with us on the edge of the sofa while we revelled in Metro-Goldwyn-Mayer carnage. He laughed at the tree as much as we did.

For a child of the 1970s, death by Dalek, werewolf, cyborg or shark was the absolute highlight of British television, the grislier the better. We knew our glee at the gore was faintly indecent, but this was celluloid make-believe, fantasy dying, and hence a permissible pleasure.

Once, though, around this time, Dad told me a story that made death – perhaps for the first time in my life – feel unnervingly close to home. My father was a physician for forty years, most of them practising as a general practitioner in an era when family doctors cared for their local community night and day, every day of the year. Before that, like his own father before him, he had sailed the high seas as a medic in the Royal Navy, and his seafaring stories transfixed me. His speciality, in my view, imbued him with the dark arts of a witch doctor. As a naval anaesthetist, he possessed the ominous power, via mysterious vapours, to 'put people to sleep' – which was, I noted, what eventually happened to my friends' pet dogs, a sleep they never woke up from.

One day, Dad began to tell me about an occasion when his naval warship was touring the South China Sea. I adored Dad's medical stories, hanging upon his every word as he told and retold, at my insistence, all my favourites. Somehow, whatever his patients threw his way – drama, trauma, poignancy, despair – Dad seemed to hold their lives in his hands with confidence, omniscience and a distinct hint of deity. He may have seen himself as only an ordinary doctor – as run of the mill, nothing special at all – but to my child's eyes he was the undisputed hero of his tales.

This story, however, was not anything like that. Dad was only a young man himself, just a few years out of medical school, when the news filtered up to his ship's sickbay that an explosion had ripped through the boiler room. Two junior ratings had been caught in the blast. 'They were even younger than me,' Dad told me. 'No more than eighteen, nineteen years old.' A faulty pressure valve had allowed a lethal build-up of steam which, when it blew, flung the lads across the room and burned most of their skin from their bodies.

'Did they die?' I asked him, unable to imagine how injuries so dramatic could be compatible with survival.

'No. At least, not to begin with. That was what made it so awful.'

Dad relayed what happened next with such absorption he forgot he was talking to a child. The two casualties were successfully dragged from the scene and rushed, still alive, to the sickbay. There, he and his senior doctor worked furiously to stabilise each patient. They dressed the burns, assessed the airways, obtained intravenous access, and started infusions of fluids and morphine.

'What's morphine?' I asked.

'A very strong painkiller. Although, in fact, they didn't need it. They were barely in pain at all.'

Knowing how excruciating mere sunburn could be, this confused me. Dad's explanation was blunt: 'You need the nerve endings in your skin to feel pain there. They didn't have any skin left, so they didn't have any nerve endings. They were pain free. Chatting, Rachel, laughing. They were full of relief. They thought they'd had a lucky escape.'

Something in the way my father said this caused me to sit up and lean closer. He was talking as though he was back there.

'We were hundreds of miles from shore. We had to sail to Hong Kong to get the lads to a hospital. It was going to take at least a day, maybe two. My job was to stay with them, comfort them. They didn't know they were dying. Why would they? They weren't in any pain. Their eyes were bandaged so they hadn't seen their injuries. But I knew. I knew that full-thickness burns over this extent of the body was fatal. I knew they'd lose consciousness long before we reached shore. My job, most of all, was to lie to them.'

The idea of professionally obligated lying had never occurred to me. As a fairly puritanical nine-year-old, I was not even sure I approved of white lies. I liked my human values rigid and polarised – right and wrong, black and white, entirely admirable and wholly unworthy. But the sadness in Dad's face, in this moment, was anything but binary. He must have ached with the knowledge, unvoiced to his patients, that one by one their organs would inexorably shut down. His voice softened as he continued talking.

'The Navy arranged to fly their parents to Hong Kong, so the boys knew – or thought they knew – that they'd be seeing their parents as soon as we arrived there. One had a girlfriend. He was worried about how he'd look to her. So I lied. I pretended they'd have a romantic reunion. I tried to make them feel positive. They hadn't been adults for very long, Rachel. To me, they still seemed not much more than children. After about twenty-four hours they started to become groggy, and not long after that they lost consciousness.'

'But ... wasn't there anything you could do to save them?' I asked.

'Nothing. Nothing at all.'

'And, then ... did they die?'

'Yes, they died, Rachel.'

Dad looked away for a moment. I wanted to cry. I was not sure what disturbed me more, the thought of the two young men sailing unknowingly to their deaths or the sight of my father, visibly overcome. Being a doctor, I had assumed, made you close to a god, and I loved having my father on that pedestal. Now I had glimpsed, even if I was unable to articulate it, the uncomfortable truth about medicine that, while the demands of the job are indeed exceptional, the person occupying the role of doctor is, just like their patients, merely human. Whether I liked it or not, I recognised my father as someone with fallibilities and frailties, just like the rest of us. And although I did not know what 'empathy' meant, I felt a little of his sadness.

None of Dad's stories lingered quite like this one. Countless times as a child I had observed his job leave him so numbed and weary on returning home to his family that he could scarcely do more than flop upon the sofa, gin and tonic in one hand, newspaper in the other. But until then I had never considered that the core of his medicine might be kindness, not heroics, and what an instinct for kindness could cost a person.

Many years later it would dawn on me that in those moments, while sweltering below deck in a windowless sick-bay, my father had in fact struggled to practise a brief and unusually horrible form of palliative medicine, the pain of which had never entirely left him. His actions that day, his lies to the two young naval ratings, were an attempt to eke out for them some quality of life, no matter how tiny, even as death bore down on them. In conventional medical terms, he had achieved nothing at all. He had not prolonged life, enhanced life, slowed death's swoop, bolstered health. Yet in human terms, by managing to stifle his horror at the charred flesh and looming demise of two young men, by keeping close at their bedsides, by ensuring they knew they were not alone, perhaps he had helped make an intolerable fate bearable. Perhaps he had done everything that mattered.

Twenty-first-century acquaintance with dying is televised, digitised, sanitised – and everywhere. My first fix of death as on-screen entertainment came courtesy of Johnny Weissmuller flexing his muscles. In the case of my son, however, it was different. At the age of eight or nine, he began returning from afternoons with his friends wired with tales of gore while anni-hilating PlayStation hordes. Forgetting the childhood frisson of seeing death at one remove, I would fret that this early exposure to make-believe gun crime would somehow bestow a blasé attitude to dying or, worse, serve to glamorize casual killing. Finn, however, put me neatly in place. He knew exactly the difference between a screen and real life: 'Er, Mum, you do know that trees aren't pixelated?'

With a doctor for a father, and a nurse for a mother, my siblings and I bucked the demographic trend for human dying to be an abstract experience. The children of medical parents often discover abnormally early that there is no neat demarcation between home and the hospital. Dad's stories were one thing. But more fundamentally, he was so immersed in his patients' lives that sometimes, unwittingly, he brought death into the home, and us out to meet it.

Once, on an idyllic Sunday afternoon, a call from the police dragged Dad away from the Ashes. All week the sun had been ferocious, the grass unmown, as an epic sporting rivalry enthralled the nation. Unusually, on this occasion, it was not the urgent need for medical expertise that denied Dad the satisfaction of watching England's cricketers thrash Australia. Instead, a bureaucratic formality was called for, one that only the on-duty doctor could provide. A few miles from our home, under milky blue skies, a young man had thrown his life into the path of a high-speed train and, as is necessary in cases of sudden or unexpected demise, a doctor was required to certify death as having occurred.

Dad had muttered as much to Mum before he departed but, as you would expect, my brother, sister and I had been kept in the dark. On his return, though, Dad's expletives were thunderous. None of us could fail to hear what had provoked them. 'Total waste of sodding time ... hardly need a bloody doctor . . . he was smeared along five hundred yards of track, for Christ's sake . . . bits of him stuck in the blackberries.'

I have no doubt I caused Dad's afternoon to deteriorate still further. 'Wait, what happened? What do you mean, "smeared"? What was in the blackberries?' My torrent of questions was relentless. Consumed with anger, which even I could tell was not entirely about missed cricket, he was forced to explain, in child-centred terms, how, even when a body has been reduced to small chunks of flesh on a track, the law still requires a doctor to diagnose and confirm death in writing.

Like his experience of tending to the two dying sailors, the event never left my father. Over the years we would revisit it, many times, in conversation. For all his appreciation of the sheer desperation that drives a person to suicide, Dad's sympathies lay with the driver, whom he had met that afternoon, on the side of the track, still trembling and retching beside his own vomit.

'In those days,' Dad told me, 'there wasn't anything like counselling or time off work for someone who went through that. You just went back to work the next day and got on with the job.'

What he never quite admitted – how could he, given what the driver had endured? – was the pain for himself, as well as for the police officers and railway staff, of being yanked from his family one weekend in late July to inspect freshly pulverised human remains beneath serenely indifferent summer skies.

What I learned as a child that Sunday was that Russians were not needed for death to strike from nowhere, suddenly and hor- ribly, and with the power to transform, if temporarily, the lives of those who had never even known the deceased, let alone of those who had loved them. One way or another we were all, I saw clearly, just moments from death. It could be folly, despair or plain bad luck – catastrophe lurked everywhere.

Dad spent the rest of the day impatient and irritable, as we cautiously gave him a wide berth. I could not conceive of doing what he did, and nor, if I were honest, did I want to.

If I thought about medicine at all as a child, it was more with ambivalence than enthusiasm. On the one hand I was addicted to Dad's tales of doctoring, but on the other, like most children, I was fully aware that doctors did things to you without permission or mercy – even my own father.

The one occasion on which I could, very easily, have died as a child was a prime example. We had driven all the way to Fort William, in the Scottish Highlands, to spend a couple of weeks in a log cabin surrounded by mountains. Old enough to be allowed to play outside by ourselves, my brother, sister and I spent hours damming streams, climbing trees and, most excitingly, swinging on a rope across a river. Except I was rubbish at rope swinging. Nervous at the prospect of falling off, I allowed my legs to trail feebly behind me, while the other children curled up tight as bullets, flinging themselves on to the other side.

As everyone issued instructions on how to do it better, slow-burning shame overtook my wimpish fear. I stood on the edge, clutching the rope with all my might, consumed by the thought that this time I had to make it to the other side. A deep breath, a moment of silence as the other children looked on like a panel of judges. Then, I launched myself into the air, wrenching my knees towards my eyeballs, determined to redeem myself.

My next sensation was of a sound worse than nails on a black-board, an ear-splitting screeching, from far away, but becoming louder and more hideous with every moment. It took a second or two before I realised the noise was coming from me. I was surprised to find myself sitting in water, submerged in it up to my neck. More baffling still was why I should be screaming when I felt neither fear nor pain. Rough hands started grabbing and clawing. My shrieks had caused adults to come sprinting from their cabins and scramble down the muddy bank to drag me up to the grass. With the hoisting and yanking came the rush of pain. I was fainting with it, too shocked and nauseous to appeal for gentleness.

Carried by my father back inside our cabin, he proceeded, as every doctor would, to conduct a brisk clinical examination. I remember Mum looking on, face pained and anxious, as Dad went straight for my right arm, now dangling at a drunken angle, to assess its range of movement. When he lifted the limb, bone ground on bone. The impact had snapped off the head of my humerus and the pain was like nothing I had known. As she watched me passing out on the sofa, Mum could not stand it any longer. 'For God's sake, Mark, stop it. Look at how much you're hurting her.'

Terse words followed, whose content I barely registered.

We set off for the nearest hospital, an hour or so away along contorted mountain roads, while I slumped on the back seat, trying in vain to keep still as the car lurched and twisted round corners. In the front, Mum and Dad discussed whether surgical fixation with metal pins would be needed, and how only an inch or two's grace had saved my neck from being broken. I kept my eyes closed, pretending to sleep, filled with gratitude to Mum for demanding that Dad take the corners a little less hastily. One surgical manipulation and a night spent driving back through the mountains later, and I endured the rest of the holiday with my arm elevated into a horizontal position by layer upon layer of dense foam packing, all kept in place by surgical tape wrapped around my torso. I looked and felt ridiculous.

The children's author Roald Dahl once told an interviewer that adults should get down on their hands and knees for a week, in order to remember what it feels like to live in a world in which all the power resides with people who literally loom over you. Nowhere are the powerlessness and indignity of being a child more evident than in a medical consultation room where you know, at any moment, you may be subjected to a spatula down your throat, a metal probe in your ear, foul-tasting liquids or a doctor's halitosis. When your parent *is* the doctor, your entire world holds those risks, even the summer holidays. It would have never occurred to me to question Dad making me faint with pain to elicit a diagnosis, had Mum not reacted against it so fiercely. But it was, I later realised, an odd quirk of fatherhood that protecting one's offspring occasionally necessitated causing them physical suffering.

Six weeks or so later, while standing in a hospital out-patients department, strip-lit and naked from the waist upwards, I received a smarting lesson in how doctors by no means monopolised the matter of pain and its infliction. My humerus had knitted together, and it was time for the foam packing and tape to be removed. I did not like the look of the nurse who grimly picked at one end of the tape, trying to dislodge it. With her severely scraped hair and thin tight mouth, to me she seemed much like a Roald Dahl antihero herself. And when she pursed her lips and prepared to pull, I was certain she did so with relish.

I gasped. The tape had adhered so tightly to my child's soft flesh that the force required for its removal took the top layer of my skin clean away. Slowly and deliberately, the nurse walked around me, tearing off translucent ribbons of skin as she went. I looked down to see beads of blood trickling towards my abdomen. Mum was aghast in the corner. I clenched my teeth, stared up into the fluorescent lights, and vowed not to make a sound, even as my eyes, swimming with tears, betrayed me.

'There,' the nurse stated, dumping bloody tape and foam into the clinical waste bin. 'That wasn't so bad, was it? I don't know what you were so worried about.'

Weeks later I still thought about her with burning hatred as I picked the old scabs off my ribcage. The fact that a centimetre here or there, a lurch to the left or a list to the right, and it could have been my neck, not my shoulder, that had snapped in two occurred to me not for a moment. Only years later would the realisation dawn that I might have been a hair's breadth from death. How innocently we all exist alongside what might have happened, yet, on this occasion, didn't.

Early clues that I might follow my father into medicine included hunting for owl pellets while walking our dog in the countryside, then spending hours dissecting out the tiny rodent bones and meticulously labelling and mounting them on cardboard. Later, when I was first taught about the female reproductive system at school, I was so appalled by the prospect of messy, embarrassing, inconvenient menstruation that I spent an entire afternoon's double biology discreetly sketching a root-and-branch pelvic redesign that diverted menstrual products from the uterus to the colon, ingeniously avoiding the unwelcome palaver of periods. As far as I was concerned, my new improved female reproductive organs beat evolution's hands down.

But as a child I did not want to be a doctor, I wanted to be a writer. I could not believe adults were given money for the pleasure of writing stories, or that you were allowed to borrow eight – eight! – books a week from the library, or that a book existed, an extraordinary book, that taught you the meanings of words. My mother describes me tearing downstairs one day and thrusting a book under her nose. 'Mum! Did you know about this book called the dictionary?' I announced ecstatically. 'It tells you what every word means *and* it even tells you how to say them.'

My own stories were obsessively transcribed, after school and at weekends, into clumsily illustrated, homemade notebooks. Gore featured prominently – disembowellings and amputations – for which I blame my father. Dad had a broom cupboard lined floor to ceiling with bookshelves. The 'library', as it was grandly known, was filled with everything from James Joyce to Harold Robbins, Isaac Asimov to Jeffrey Archer. From early childhood, I surreptitiously devoured age-inappropriate fodder, continuing late at night with a torch beneath the duvet, long after Mum and Dad had gone to bed themselves. The James Bond and Modesty Blaise series were best for racy excitement, while the horrors of Edgar Allan Poe both repelled and enthralled me, inspiring my own gruesome dramas.

The best stories, of course, came not from a book but from Dad himself. Dr Mark Rendall came to know intimately many generations of patients — all the loves, losses, hardships and joys that knit families together, or sometimes tear them apart. He could not walk down the street of the little market town where he practised without a string of cheery hellos called out to Dr Rendall. At Christmas, there were so many gift-wrapped bottles from grateful patients we could not fit them all under the tree.

From his children's perspective, all of this meant nothing. Time spent devoted to the needs of his patients meant time away from us, and from Mum. Often, like so many doctors, Dad returned home at the end of the day as empty and spent as a field after harvest. Having poured all of himself into back-to-back consultations, there was nothing left for his family. The innocuous-sounding 'one in three' — his standard GP's roster — had to be lived to be believed. Every third day of his working life, he worked thirty-six hours straight, from nine in the morning until six or seven o'clock the following evening. All night long, patients would call him out on visits to their homes. Mum answered the telephone calls while Dad was out responding to them, so both my parents suffered semi-permanent sleep deprivation. Sometimes, after a particularly gruelling night, as Dad helped us get ready for school in the morning, he looked so haggard and worn that even making coffee seemed beyond him, let alone another day spent making potentially life-and-death decisions with patients. Fatigue quickened his temper as we fumbled with schoolbags and shoes, dragging our feet in the hall.

Once a year I glimpsed for myself the clinical world that claimed so much of my father. Every Christmas, my siblings and I would rip open the contents of our stockings and devour

our special festive breakfast before setting off for Dad's local cottage hospital in the car with my parents. These small, rural hospitals, now largely closed down, enabled villagers to avoid huge treks to a county hospital, and to be treated close to home by the one doctor, their local general practitioner, who was familiar with their life and problems. Babies were born there, great-grandparents died there. My father knew every one of them.

Each year, a handful of his patients, men and women in their eighties or their nineties, would spend Christmas marooned in the cottage hospital. Dad moved from bedside to bedside, chatting warmly and easily, with his young family in tow. At barely five or six years old, I would hover uneasily at each ancient patient's side, nauseated by the smells of iodine and bodily fluids. Rarely was anyone else there. Sometimes, it seemed as though the visit from the family doctor was the highlight, so far, of their Christmas Day.

For all my anxieties about what to say, how to behave and whether someone was about to gasp their terminal breath in front of me, one thing was clear. These faces, so wizened and old, would light up with delight at my father's arrival. And when my siblings and I crept closer to their sides, often they would beam with joy at the chance to chat with a small child. Somehow I knew that in spite of my fears and awkwardness, the little we gave of our Christmas mornings mattered greatly to my father's bedbound patients.

By the time it came for me to choose my A-levels, medicine felt no more connected to people than school chemistry did to medicine. Except for Dad. He was the link. He made medicine human. As I had grown up, the stories I had once loved for the way they framed Dad as my two-dimensional childhood hero had become a nuanced, complicated and treasured form of father-daughter intimacy. When we talked about his patients, he shared himself with me, the reserved, self-questioning doctor who wore his losses and failures – his patients' deaths – like rust around his heart. For the first time, it crossed my mind that perhaps, all those years ago, when Dad had manipulated my broken arm, it had hurt him as much as me to do so.

'Dad, you know if I do English A-level it means I can't do Chemistry?'

We were chatting one Sunday morning while walking the dog through the farmland that surrounded our house. The deadline for me to submit my A-level choices loomed the next day. My sixth form was small, and Chemistry clashed with English on the timetable. Dad knew exactly what this signified.

'So, if you choose the subject that's essential for Medicine, you won't be able to study the one you love more than anything?'

I nodded. We walked on. The silence hung comfortably between us. Some way in the distance, our Labrador was chasing rabbits with such inept enthusiasm that we both burst out laughing. We stomped through the mud, skirting the cowpats. I hesitated before asking the question I knew my father would not answer.

'Dad . . . do you think I should be a doctor?'

Had he said yes, I would have followed his lead in an instant, and he was, I knew, well aware of that. He paused, then smiled. 'I can't tell you what to be, Rachel. Only you know that.'

Not once, to their credit, had either of my parents ever tried to steer me towards their vision of the life that was best for me. I knew how grateful I should be for that, yet still longed for Dad to tell me what to do. In the end, ironically, it was because of him that I ruled out a career in medicine by choosing to study books above Bunsen burners. I was wary of becoming a doctor not out of genuine vocation but instead, deep down, to make him proud of me.

Rather than helping people through healing, I harboured instead a vague, romantic, childish notion of using words to make the world a better place. Stories, I knew, were infinitely more than mere entertainment. Not only could stories save lives, but people sometimes died trying to tell them. As an idealistic teenager, I watched transfixed as the BBC broadcast images from China's Tiananmen Square of a thin man in shirt sleeves standing in front of a dictatorship's tanks, defying them to crush him as the world's press looked on. The idea that speaking out, of telling the truth, could easily, in another part of the world, end up being the death of you made journalism seem like a moral imperative. Through all those years hanging on tenterhooks as Dad enthralled me with his tales of doctoring, it never occurred to me that the heart of both jobs, journalism and medicine, might fundamentally be storytelling.

I gave neither medicine nor mortality another thought until, just before setting off for university – Philosophy, Politics and Economics my degree of choice – I was forced to confront, in a rush of adrenalin, the apparent fact that I was about to die.

It was deep winter, one of those dismal English days in which dawn never properly breaks and by teatime, the dregs of daylight are gone. My friend in the village had plans though. Tom rocked up on the doorstep that evening, hardly able to stand still as he spun a battered set of car keys from his fingertips. 'It's mine, all mine,' he boasted eagerly. 'Fancy a spin?'

I gawped at the banger on the driveway. To me, these superannuated wheels promised more thrills than the world's fastest Ferrari. A car – any car – was a means of escape from the back of beyond. Pure intoxication.

'Wait. Is this actually yours? Have your parents really given you a car?' I gasped.

Tom had passed his driving test a few days earlier. His reward, from his parents, was deliciously unexpected. 'Yep. Come on. Let's go.'

There are no surprises as to how this story ends. It was bitterly cold, with frost in the air. Black ice had been daubing the country lanes all week. After a stuttering start and some amateur reversing, we crept sedately through the village at a law-abiding pace and then, out in the open, began to accelerate. Tom whooped as he crunched through the gears. There was a wildness about his desire for speed that initially did not frighten me. We laughed together as the engine strained and spluttered, and the hedgerows began to melt away around us. The speed, the liberation, as we played at being grown-ups, claiming the roads as our own.

But Tom's first taste of speed had unleashed something primal and dangerous. With his foot to the floor, the engine first roared, then screamed in protest. I began to bristle with fear. 'Hey, Tom. You need to slow down.' It was as though I had not spoken. 'Tom, seriously, slow down. You're going too fast. Tom!' The more I begged, the more recklessly he swerved. My screams only seemed to incite him.

Even as adrenalin flooded my body – my panic a kind of bile in my mouth – a part of me observed the road ahead with cold, hard, unflinching clarity. I knew, with utter certainty, how the next seconds would play out. Tom's shaky hold on the tarmac was about to fracture. The car would no longer be swerving but skidding. He would fight for control and never regain it. We would be flung into oncoming traffic. The shriek of wheels, the smash of cranium on glass, would go unfelt, unnoticed, because moments from now we would be mangled and lifeless, dangling inertly from our seatbelts.

And sure enough, the car began to lurch from one lane to the next. Tom's wrenching on the steering wheel was futile. I could not tell if the thundering in my head was my blood or the brake pads on metal. Neither of us could change how this would end now. When we were flung, for the third time, into the opposite lane, the car had acquired such drunken momentum that its wheels left the road – we were launched skywards. A thud, a screech, the crumpling of metal and then we were upside down in a ditch, axles spinning above us.

Every window was smashed, the bodywork chewed up, the car a write-off. No one could have crawled from that wreckage intact, yet somehow we emerged, coated head to toe in glass, scratched and trembling but otherwise unscathed. We stood on the road next to smoking scrap metal, silently clutching each other. It was bitterly cold. Our breaths, condensed, were visible proof to the world and ourselves that we were still, against all odds, alive.

On the far side of the road was a country cottage, outside

which an elderly woman stood in her nightie. 'Come here,' she called, leading us inside. "The bang woke me up. I thought there'd been an explosion.'

I borrowed her telephone to call my parents for help, shards of glass from my hair pattering on to the table. Mum and Dad arrived, stared in horror at the wreckage, and drove us home in silence. What was there, really, to say? Tom and I never spoke of what had happened. And, after a day or so of intrusive, slow-motion, high-definition replays, I successfully dismissed the crash from my mind. *Move along,* I told myself. *Do not stop, do not look back. You are eighteen years old and there is all this life to be living.*

2

Flesh and Blood

They come to rest at any kerb:
All streets in time are visited.

Philip Larkin, 'Ambulances'
from *The Whitsun Weddings*

The first time I saw a dead body, I would be lying if I pretended I'd cared.

It is spring, but the city is giddy with the audacity of summer. Now in my mid-twenties, I have lived in London long enough to know that unseasonal bursts of rare British sunshine bring out the capital's carnival spirit. During those fleeting moments of snatched not-quite summer, the hard edges of life in the city – noses crushed into armpits on tube trains, altercations between drivers over who hogged the road – melt away as we turn our heads skywards, like plants to the light, marvelling at the blueness and warmth.

On Friday 30 April 1999, the frayed tempers and short fuses of an overcrowded metropolis vanish beneath limitless skies. I am a young television journalist who occasionally indulges a secret pipedream of retraining, one day, as a doctor. By the time I leave the studios that evening with my boyfriend, London has been dipped in gold. Coats off, smiles on, we saunter slowly across Hungerford Bridge, taking our time to savour the light rebounding off the Thames beneath us. We are searching for a pub outside which we can sit to toast this improbable gift of an evening. It seems the whole of London has had the same idea. The streets of Soho teem with young men and women spilling out on to the pavements, pints in hand.

Arm in arm with Matt, semi-intoxicated ourselves with sunshine, I find myself marvelling at the transformative power of something as simple as weather. In place of the hard-bitten commuters, clawing their individual ways home for the week-end, it feels like London has come together in humble worship of the sun.

We weave towards a pub that happens to be located in Soho's Old Compton Street, the heart of London's LGBT community. I like the Admiral Duncan. A small but vibrant gay bar, packed with personality. Its swagger and attitude reflect many of its customers. But this evening, unbeknown to us all, somebody wants them dead.

When it happens, we are approaching the pub's front door. I have no recollection of the actual blast, only of finding myself face down in the gutter. My cheeks are pressed against tarmac. A forest of legs looms above. Although perplexed, I am oddly unmoved by how the street has lurched on its axis, been upended around me, and I can no longer hear a sound.

Slowly I stand, stunned and silent, wondering why the people around me are coated in dust as thick as flour. Of my five senses, only my eyes seem to function. A few feet in front of me lies a body in the gutter. Dimly, I clock how bright the man's blood is, and that his leg, neatly severed, lies on the ground beside him. The street is flooded with his blood. Other people, I notice, are wandering in circles, ghosts with neither purpose nor direction. I survey them idly, feeling nothing. I cannot remember why I am there.

Suddenly, police officers are everywhere, screaming at us all to get back, though I can tell this only from their contorted expressions, still unable to hear. We are herded at pace away from the scene. I acquiesce, allowing myself to be shunted backwards, baffled by why the police are so frantic, unable to run as they demand.

In the mêlée, I happen to come across Matt, about whom I have completely forgotten, and we set off, wordlessly, across London. In place of conversation is the weight of the unspoken as we walk and walk for aimless miles. Perhaps we are hoping that if we put enough distance between ourselves and the blast we will somehow make it unhappen. At some stage, I start to shake. We have to halt for a while so I do not fall over. Several hours after the attack we find ourselves back in our flat in London's East End. Ears still ringing, we sit glued to the television, transfixed by the coverage of the explosion that nearly killed us. Another second, another footstep, a purposeful stride in place of our meander. It is only then, late at night, staring at the footage of the chaos we have just left, that I start to feel properly frightened – or, indeed, anything at all.

The facts, as they emerge in the media, are bleak. Three people were killed – one of them a pregnant woman – and more than eighty others injured when the device, a nail bomb, tore through the Admiral Duncan. One man was blown thirty feet into the air by the force of the blast. Was this the man I had seen before me, cleaved, desecrated, lying in a pool of his own blood? The pages and pages of print make me queasy. As a journalist myself, I am acutely aware that nothing makes good copy quite like other people's misery. Still, I cannot stop reading.

The nail bomber, a white supremacist called David Copeland, exploded three devices in total, deliberately targeting the black, Bengali and gay communities of Brixton, Brick Lane and Soho respectively. At his trial, he declares himself a righteous messenger from God, hailing his nail bomb campaign as the start of a long-overdue homophobic and race war. Convicted for murder, he is sentenced to serve six consecutive, resolutely secular, life sentences in prison.

In the weeks that follow the bombing, my dreams take a nightmarish turn. It seems that all the fear I did not feel at the time is, one way or another, going to force its way out. I never discuss it with anyone, but at night I sometimes wake up in panic, gasping for air; then, during the day, I feel preoccupied with guilt at how I did nothing for the victims around me. The man with no leg, the dead and dying. It had not occurred to me to try and help any of them. You could put this down to shock, but I know that the truth is, even had I been in a state to help others, I would not have really known how to.

Twenty-one ambulances and one air ambulance did help that evening, delivering their crews of paramedics and doctors into, not away from, the danger – in order to keep people like me from harm. Scores of policemen and women did the same. Did death cross their minds, or only duty? None of these hundreds of first responders knew at the time whether there was one bomb, or more blasts to come. In racing to the scene and evacuating the public to safety, they were, depending on your point of view, merely getting on with their jobs or behaving as consummate heroes. Perhaps a modern-day superhero is precisely that, a jobbing, ordinary bloke or woman who, when the situation demands it, steps up without a moment's pause – squarely ignoring their own vulnerability – and risks their own life to save others.

At age twenty-five, outside the Admiral Duncan pub that day, I discovered that the digitised death that surrounds us daily – in all its cartoon, games console or multiplex varieties – prepares us not a jot for the haunting reality of flesh and blood, actual dying. For nearly two decades I dealt with the first human corpse I ever confronted by pretending to myself I had not in fact seen it. The idea that a man had bled to his death before my eyes while I limply looked on, doing nothing, was too painful properly to acknowledge. I chose, instead, denial.

This early brush with death was, then, typical of my age and our time. Although older adults usually experience protracted periods of ill health and decline – in which the boundary between living and dying becomes blurred, indistinct, and can sometimes span years – in twenty-first-century Britain, sudden or violent deaths and near misses are the most common mode of dying for the young. Road traffic collisions account for over 60 per cent of childhood deaths in the UK, for example. And when, like a thunderbolt or the wrath of God, death strikes instantaneously, there is no time to talk or plan. You are felled before you know what is happening.

Such proximity to dying at the random hands of a nail

bomber only cemented my conviction that death denial was sensible. There was little advantage in morbidly brooding on my possible demise when no amount of speculation could prevent it. I could, for sure, become neurotic and fretful, but how much better to *live*, grabbing each moment, inhabiting them wisely. Who knew, after all, how many I would be granted. As for dwelling on my distant future descent into old age, that seemed like the height of self-indulgence. I knew that my body, still bursting with energy and vigour, would one day wither and decay into something stooped and enfeebled, a husk of the physical form I took now. But why would I wish to contemplate ageing and dying, as a creature hardwired to live? I had evaded death twice now. I had defied her. She was not coming for me.

Many years later, the Soho nail bombing cropped up over breakfast with a friend, a consultant in trauma anaesthesia at St Mary's Hospital, London, one of the capital's major trauma centres. Helgi Johannsson specialises in confronting what terrorists leave behind. To a doctor, trauma is not, primarily, distress or anguish but the physical affront of bullet through flesh, car across limb, metal into skull, crushed chest beneath rubble. Trauma teams attend to the bolts from the blue – bodily injuries of such swiftness and severity that they may, unless instantly stabilised, deprive their hosts of life before they ever have a chance to feel traumatised.

Helgi deals on a daily basis with the kind of mangled, twisted, broken bodies that make even other doctors quail, let alone the non-medically trained. Sudden, shocking, brutal death is his bread and butter. He told me he stopped being scared of terrorist activity a long time ago. This is not because

London is besieged by acts of terror but because personal tragedy of unimaginable order – lives torn apart with neither reason
nor warning – comprises his ordinary day at the office.

'I treat people who just happened to be in the wrong place
at the wrong time,' he said. 'You learn how arbitrary and
precarious life is. Once, I heard a nurse telling my patient, a
young woman who had been stabbed nearly to death by her
partner, that there was a reason for what had happened to her,
a meaning to it. I said, "No, that's just the random shittiness of
life." The patient liked that – she really laughed. I truly believe
that though. We live in a random world where anything can
happen at any moment, but it's full of beauty and goodness too.'

He paused to relish a mouthful of toast. It was hard to believe
that this clear-eyed physician, who regards terrorists as no more
of a threat than the infinite cruelty of acts of chance, had ever
faced death without equanimity. But even Helgi once baulked
at confronting the dying. We discovered, while chatting, to
our mutual astonishment, that he too was in Old Compton
Street on the day David Copeland unleashed his hate there. A
young doctor himself then, only a couple of years out of medical school, Helgi instinctively sprinted towards the carnage in
which I had numbly floundered.

'I probably ran straight past you,' he told me. 'The risks
didn't cross my mind for a second. Things like secondary
devices weren't even a consideration, I just ran to help. But I
was completely out of my comfort zone. I was completely inexperienced. I had no real idea how to deal with the casualties. I
had no equipment whatsoever. And, as you know, you're stark
bollock naked without your equipment as a doctor. You're so
limited. I got members of the public wrapping up bleeding

limbs and doing compressions on chests until the paramedics arrived. But I felt utterly helpless.'

I had often wondered whether my own impotence that day, a private source of shame, had triggered a resolve to retrain as a doctor. For Helgi, this early encounter with trauma – one for which he felt wholly unprepared – went on to shape his subsequent career. 'I hated the helplessness, being unable to do more at the scene. I dealt with that by deciding there and then to go into anaesthesia, and acquire some proper skills, so that never again would I feel that helpless as a doctor.'

Our conversation allowed me to lay a demon to rest. 'Was he real?' I asked Helgi. 'The man with no leg? I'm sure I saw a man with no leg – it was lying on the ground beside him. Was he real?'

Yes, came the answer. Entirely, indisputably real. No figment of a shocked imagination. A young man, full of life, drink in hand, enjoying an uncanny foray by summer into springtime, butchered in his prime.

It is hard, but salutary, to imagine inhabiting an era in which choosing to ignore our inevitable demise is not an option because sudden, shocking, fatal acts of chance are ubiquitous, felling young and old alike. When the eighteenth-century philosopher Thomas Hobbes famously described the human condition as 'nasty, brutish and short', he was referring specifically to the state of mankind prior to the formation of central government, a perpetual war of all against all. But to me, the description always struck deeper. Sure, a state apparatus could hold in check the worst of human nature, but it took the advent of modern medicine to liberate us from the infections, diseases, accidents and sheer bad luck that used to snuff us out, in droves, in our prime.

Less than a century ago, for example, my maternal grandmother, Nessie, lived in an area of Glasgow notorious for its urban deprivation. In 1925, more than two decades before Britain created its national health service, Nessie was a girl of ten or eleven. Four children, their mother and father were squeezed into a tiny two-room tenement with no electricity, running water or indoor toilet. The outdoor privy was shared by five, maybe six more families. In spite of owning next to nothing, Nessie's mother − my great-grandmother − never failed to keep the two rooms spotless.

Invalided on the battlefields of the First World War, Nessie's father was unable to work, and 1920s Depression Britain was no time for a poor family to be without its male breadwinner. Mammy made ends meet by sewing piecework garments late into the night by candlelight. Annie, the oldest child, had already been helping her stitch for years. There was barely enough money for food, let alone savings set aside for a doctor's visit that might easily cost a week and a half's wages.

One night, the two girls, Nessie and Annie, were huddled, unobserved, on a threadbare mattress, conversing in urgent whispers.

'What is it, Annie, what's wrong?' asked Nessie.

'It's my belly,' she said, face flushed and damp with sweat. 'A bad pain.'

'Shall I tell Mammy?' asked Nessie, alarmed at her fifteen-year-old sister's discomfort.

'No. No, you can't tell her. She'll worry. We can't afford the doctor anyway.'

Nessie, by nature a timid little girl, had always deferred to her older sister, and did not dare defy her now, however distressing she found the sight of Annie gritting her teeth with pain. She reached out to squeeze her sister's palm, anxiety knotting her stomach.

Annie turned to the wall and lay as still as she could beneath the blankets. The slightest movement was excruciating. Slowly, the evening wore on. By the time her three siblings clambered into bed beside her, Annie found their slightest shuffle almost unbearably painful. It took great effort of will not to cry out, and even more not to ask for her mother.

The 1920s were a time of extraordinary medical innovation. Breakthroughs included the discovery of penicillin and of insulin, the first vaccines against measles and tuberculosis, and the use of iron lungs to prevent patients infected with polio from suffocating. Yet a doctor's attention was no basic essential, but a luxury – dispensed, primarily, to those who could pay. All over Britain there were thousands of impoverished families who would never know a doctor's care for want of the means to purchase it.

Mammy rubbed her eyes, put her piecework to one side, and was asleep the moment she crawled beneath the blankets, unaware that in the bed next door her eldest child lay rigid and wakeful. Pain ebbed and flowed in the darkness. Annie's appendix was angry, inflamed, throbbing with infection, yet she endured her suffering in silence.

Time crawled. At some stage during the night the pressure grew too great and her appendix burst, flooding her abdomen with pus. Maybe the other children in the bed heard their big sister muttering and rambling as overwhelming sepsis induced a delirium. By the time dawn broke, Annie lay outstretched and cold, dead beside her siblings.

Only very recently, long after my grandmother had herself died, did my mother tell me this story. I was stunned, dumbfounded. You might imagine the most shocking thing about the tale to be the notion of a child electing to endure fatal levels of pain rather than worry her parents with the revelation of an illness for which they could not afford to call a doctor. But it was not. It was what came next.

'Imagine waking up to find your own sister, a child, lying dead in bed beside you. It must have been so traumatic,' I had said to Mum.

Patiently, Mum exhaled. 'I think Nessie probably just accepted it, to be honest.' She paused. 'That's just how it was in those days.'

This took time to sink in. Cosseted by twenty-first-century creature comforts, safe in the knowledge that my loved ones had high-quality healthcare to rely on, I ruminated on what Mum had told me. My own children, at the time, were ten and six. The idea of my oldest, Finn, waking up to find his little sister, Abbey, dead in the bed beside him was appalling enough, let alone that of him being so inured to dying, so exposed to random death, that he would take such a horror in his stride.

But there it was. In Britain, less than a century ago, death in the home was so frequent, so commonplace, that family members regarded the witnessed loss of their loved ones as entirely expected – as normal. What seems to us today a violation, a horror, was just the way it was back then.

*

Being a young, enthusiastic documentary-maker in one of the most vibrant cities in the world was a heady experience for a sheltered twentysomething from deepest rural Wiltshire. Television in those days was fuelled by free-flowing alcohol and small mountains of cocaine. I was surrounded by clever, savvy, urbane folk who could talk virtually anyone into doing anything. Power rested predominantly in the hands of older men, some of whom were predatory, targeting their youngest female colleagues such as me. Once, an entire production team of which I was a member was invited by the boss to a country retreat. We strolled around the grounds, champagne flutes in hand, wittily – as we saw it – dissecting the state of the nation. My boss beckoned me over to a statue on the lawn.

'Look at her, Rachel, what does she remind you of?'

We were alone, cut off from the rest of the party, and I was, I suppose, twenty-two or twenty-three. I stared down at a stone sculpture of a nubile young woman, lying belly down at my feet. Her back was arched, her face tilted backwards, while a fountain tinkled on to the small of her back, like an eternal al fresco ejaculation. As I tried in vain to think of an answer, the boss supplied one for me.

'Do you know, Rachel, I'll tell you who she reminds me of,' he murmured, while caressing her natal cleft with his barefoot toe. 'She reminds me of you.'

You always hope you will come up with a devastating riposte in these scenarios, but they are mortifying, cheapening and, more than anything, diminishing. I smiled weakly, not wanting to appear impolite, even while cursing myself for not punching him.

Journalism and I were a queasy fit. Obsessive by nature, prone to rampant perfectionism, I would lose myself completely in every documentary I made, then come up for air, six months lost to a film, feeling hollowed out, pared to the bone. Mum achieved a lifelong ambition when she was awarded a degree from the Open University. But I was not there at her graduation, because I was ingratiating myself with warlords in central Africa to capture footage of Congolese child soldiers. The end justified the means, I told myself – in this case, we would bring a barely covered civil war to the screen – but the means were long and lonely, and too often entailed the relegation of loved ones. I was the friend who let you down at the last minute, the one you could not be certain would turn up in a crisis, the flaky, insubstantial one, careering from story to story, wondering why the good one could do through responsible journalism so often, day to day, felt so bad.

Slowly, insidiously, as the months went by, this hollowness became pathological. One day, the morning after my latest documentary had been broadcast, I lay in the tub, tears dripping into bathwater, each plaudit and celebratory message stoking panic, not pride. The thought of going through it again, fighting tooth and nail to try and tell a story faultlessly, was unbearable. I was shocked to find myself daydreaming about ways of ending my life, and immediately reached for Dad.

'Hey,' I muttered flatly on the end of the phone.

'Oh hello, Rachel,' came the reassuring reply.

He told me about the garden, his recent walks through the fields, the return, as every springtime, of the skylarks above. Mum was learning bridge, Dad was irate at something Tony Blair had done, they were planning a trek through the mountains of Corsica. Life, in all its banality and glory, comfortably ticking along.

'What's wrong?' he asked, after a while.

'I'm tired,' I answered quietly. 'Really tired.'

A pause. They were always easy between us. He waited for me to go on.

'I love being a journalist, but . . . it's hard and . . . and sometimes I think I made a mistake . . . Maybe I would have been happier if I'd been a doctor.'

'I think you would be an excellent doctor, Rachel.' I noted the tense, future not past, as though somehow this might be a realisable prospect.

'Do you? Do you really, Dad?'

Although I did not believe him, the idea still felt like a lifeline. But I was too burned-out to work for a while and went into hiding instead, ostensibly trying to figure out a future, though in reality buried beneath my duvet and depression, scarcely leaving the flat.

In the end, the best I could come up with was this. Journalism, for all its excitement and power – a reach of millions of people each time a programme was broadcast – might have been the dream job on paper, but it gnawed away at my soul. Ingratiation felt shabby. I did not want to persuade, entice or manipulate anyone into appearing on camera. If I were going to work this hard, this all-consumingly, at something it needed to feel cleaner, more straightforward. And it simply could not be this difficult. I knew about imposter syndrome, and that this permanent sense of fraudulence was probably more to do with me than journalism – but how could I be certain without trying something else first? When you are lying in the bath and images of slitting your own wrists float into your mind, at least you have nothing to lose.

I wish I could pretend my decision to retrain as a doctor was some blinding epiphany of vocation and selflessness, but it was more of a scrambled retreat from an intolerable present, a parachute from the here and now. I was trying to save myself, not other people, and so, shamefaced, I concealed my true motives from everyone, even my father.

Turning a pipedream into a place at medical school entailed hauling myself back to work while moonlighting at night on my missing science A-levels. To my surprise, my half-baked plan, for all the desperation that preceded its conception, proved to be an antidote against sinking back into depression. I cared that little bit less about crafting stories for television, and found that caring less made the crafting easier. I could breathe again. And I discovered, to my astonishment, that chemistry, when studied at the age of twenty-eight, was nothing short of intoxicating. The idea that the behaviour of every solid, liquid, gas and living thing could be pared down to the basic chemical properties of the 118 elements of the Periodic Table – and, more specifically, to the number of electrons orbiting their nuclei – had an elegance and power that took my breath away. Every chemical reaction of the human body boiled down to this – gyrating specks in graceful orbits, interacting as predicted by the textbook on my desk at home. It was beautiful, magical, thrilling. An epiphany of sorts – the bewitchery of science.

Securing a place at university, on the other hand, was a tactical exercise. I dutifully bought the expensive guidebooks on how to win that coveted place at medical school, scouring them from cover to cover to ascertain the best strategy for interview and application form. Apparently, much like the ingratiation expected by war criminals, medical school interview panels required their subjects to jump through all manner of hoops that signalled 'doctor material'. One diktat was particularly strident: do not, under any circumstances, even consider admitting that your motivation for studying medicine was a desire to help people. God forbid, the books implied, you should say anything so crass and naive. The moment you whispered the H-word, you would be kissing goodbye to dreams of stethoscopes for ever.

Despite my newfound obsession with seeing people in terms of orbiting electrons, I read this advice with consternation. It seemed to me that these books, written by practising doctors, were sending a less than subtle message to sixth formers everywhere that their instinct to help others was something to hush up, a clandestine failing that risked incurring the wrath of the gatekeepers to a supposedly caring profession. Even before setting foot in a medical school they were somehow being groomed that talking openly and sincerely about their true motivations could diminish their prospects as a doctor.

When it came to my own interviews, I knew that being an applicant at least a decade older than the rest, with an unusual current career in television, was going to provoke particular interest in my motives. I could not quite bring myself to full disclosure. 'This is my idiosyncratic strategy for evading a relapse into suicidal depression' did not quite convey the impression of a safe pair of hands. But I could be truthful about the other things that drove me. And helping people – wanting to do something good for others – was, and always had been, a powerful impulse.

Somewhat surreally, I found myself sitting in front of a panel of professors behind which, stranded in formaldehyde, was an array of human body parts in jars. Ears, brains, eye-balls, hearts and other, more ominous, fillets of flesh, which I fervently hoped I would not be asked to identify. 'Is this the first test of doctoring?' I wondered. 'To manage to answer coherently a question from a professor who is inches away from an embalmed human liver?' None of us mentioned the anatomy specimens. I was being watched by a pickled eyeball that everyone pretended was not there. A more macabre admission interview I could not imagine.

'So, tell us, Rachel, what made you decide to study medicine?' someone asked.

'Well,' I answered, refusing to game this, 'I know you're not supposed to say that you want to be a doctor because you want to help people, but the truth is, I do. That's what it comes down to. I could come up with all kinds of clever alternative reasons, but the fact is, I want to go to work each day and do something decent and good, that I can take pride in, and I think that should be the essence of medicine.'

Polite smiles all round. And then, quick as a flash: 'That's very interesting. But tell us, what's it like working in ... television?'

'Oh. Well, television is all about people too, in a fundamental sense. It's about building relationships with people, ensuring they can trust you, then trying to tell a human story as effectively as you can.' I even tried to articulate the bits I found challenging, like the risk, always present, that you might inadvertently exploit someone.

At each university, the interview was the same, dominated by intrigue about television. What was it like, had I met people who were famous, why would I want to leave a job like that?

'Tell us,' said one interviewer, 'what's it like working with Jon Snow? Is he as nice in real life as he seems to be on *Channel 4 News*?'

'Look,' I wanted to say, 'enough about the bloody television. Can't we, you know, discuss electrons or something?'

I knew I had got in. The television clinched it. When I called home to tell my parents the news, I could hear the smile in Dad's voice. Those words, said with utmost sincerity: 'I'm very proud of you, Rachel.'

3

Skirting Death

Death is not the opposite of life, but a part of it.

Haruki Murakami, 'Firefly', *Blind Willow,
Sleeping Woman: 24 Stories*

It started reasonably enough. The clean-cut, efficient young doctor explaining to the fifty-year-old woman in a hospital gown that he needed to conduct an internal examination. Unflinching, she held her shaved head high.

'I guess we'll start the exam,' said Dr Jason Posner. 'Why don't you just sort of lie back and relax. Won't take a minute.'

There can be no dignity in placing your feet up high in gynaecological stirrups, but Vivian Bearing has been living with Stage 4 ovarian cancer. Indignity has dogged her for some time.

Stoically, she eyeballed the fluorescent lights, preparing to surrender her body, once again, to her doctors. It was then that commonplace indignity twisted into something more unpleasant. Vivian's doctor had forgotten that an intimate examination required a chaperone – to protect both patient and clinician from the possibility of inappropriate touching.

'I've got to go get Susie,' an exasperated Jason muttered. 'I've got to have a girl here – some crazy clinical rule.'

He exited the room to find the nurse in question, leaving Vivian alone, still strung up in stirrups, her exposure absolute. As the seconds crawled by, she tried to distract herself by chanting first her times tables, then metaphysical poetry in her head. When, finally, the doctor returned, she had been waiting, laid out like a specimen upon a slab, for what had felt like a forever of shame.

'Why did you leave her like this?' asked Susie, horrified.

'I had to find you,' answered Jason, brusquely. 'Now come on.' His internal examination was thorough to the point of brutality. Afterwards, Vivian commented drily: 'One thing that can be said for an eight-month course of cancer treatment: it is highly educational. I am learning to suffer.'

Vivian, mercifully, is fictitious, though one senses she is rooted in real women's experiences. Her creator, the American playwright Margaret Edson, used to work in an oncology department. In 1999, she was awarded the Pulitzer Prize for her drama *Wit*, widely regarded as the best play ever written about cancer.

On my very first day at medical school I was shown the film version of *Wit*, starring the actress Emma Thompson. Three hundred of us trotted innocently into the lecture hall, the vast majority still teenagers, fresh out of school. We were intrigued that a movie, of all things, had been deemed sufficiently important to occupy the first afternoon of our medical school timetables. I later realised that whoever in the faculty had decided to inaugurate our learning in this manner was an educational genius. We were about to be hit with a celluloid sledgehammer.

Vivian Bearing is a fiercely intelligent American professor specialising in the sonnets of the seventeenth-century metaphysical poet John Donne. Upon diagnosis with late-stage ovarian cancer, she is admitted to a New York teaching hospital to undergo gruelling treatment with experimental trial drugs. From the outset, the play captures superbly the loss of control patients typically feel upon admission to hospital, as we are stripped, gowned, prodded and scrutinised by a doctorly elite that holds all the power.

As a research subject, Vivian is particularly vulnerable. Even her supposedly informed consent to untested treatments is undone by her consultant's insistence that in exchange for his trial drugs she must withstand whatever side effects are inflicted upon her.

'The important thing is for you to take the full dose of chemotherapy,' he coerces her. 'There may be times when you wish for a lesser dose, due to the side effects. But we've got to go full force.'

To her doctors, Vivian is less a human being than research fodder. Their route to publication in a prestigious journal, perhaps – if only she yields decent results. Even when the therapeutic benefits are doubtful, her team continues to urge her to submit to eye-watering doses of chemotherapy, driven more by a hunger for data than a thirst for healing. In her sterile, strip-lit ward, we witness Vivian endure the inevitable side effects – severe vomiting, pain and humiliation. She becomes acutely aware that her body is now, to her medical team, what

Donne's sonnets used to be to her – an object, to be probed and interrogated ruthlessly in order, at best, to further academic understanding or, at worst, her doctors' own careers.

In withering asides, Vivian deconstructs her hospital experience with the same rigour she might have applied to a sonnet. After being used by her consultant to teach students one morning, she turns to the camera and comments archly:

> *In grand rounds they read me like a book.*
> *Once I did the teaching . . .*
> *Now I am taught.*
> *This is much easier,*
> *I just hold still and look cancerous.*

For the whole hundred minutes of *Wit* we felt pinned to our seats in painful silence. Though I knew the play was to some extent a caricature, more relevant to the medicine of a bygone era, the idea that any doctor could treat their patients so callously was deeply uncomfortable. I was a starry-eyed enthusiast that day, longing to dive unthinkingly into my medical textbooks. *Wit* drew me up short. It compelled me to consider my future power as a doctor – my potential to dehumanise, distress and even hurt my patients. For an audience of neophyte medics, the film was, in short, the best possible medicine. It forced us to see ourselves through our future patients' eyes, and to confront our capacity to wound.

But there was more that mattered on screen. In five long years of medical school, watching *Wit*, I would discover in retrospect, was the one – the only – occasion during which as a student I was ever invited to consider human mortality.

Like Donne before her – whose poems are fiendishly cerebral meditations on death's inevitability, bursting with intricate conceits and paradoxes – Vivian confronts her terror of dying with an arsenal of cleverness and wit. She intellectualises her imminent demise, using irony and humour to deflect the visceral horrors she knows are to come. Yet the words that have served her so well throughout life become increasingly hollow as life begins quietly to dispose of her.

'Now is not the time for verbal swordplay,' she states bluntly after a frank discussion with Susie, her nurse, about whether she would wish for CPR in the event that her heart stopped beating:

> *Nothing would be worse than a detailed scholarly analysis and*
> *Erudition, interpretation, complication.*
> *No. Now is the time for simplicity.*
> *Now is the time for, dare I say it, kindness.*
> *And I thought being extremely smart would take care of it.*
> *But I see that I have been found out.*
> *I'm scared.*

In one of the play's most moving scenes, Vivian's old professor from her undergraduate days, the fearsomely intellectual E. M. Ashford, pays an unexpected visit to her former student. Despite her reputation as a merciless scholar, Ashford immediately grasps not only that Vivian is dying, but that she needs, in this moment, nothing more than simple kindness. Instinctively, she curls her elderly frame up on to the bed next to Vivian, as a mother might comfort her feverish child, and begins to read aloud from the picture book she has just bought her great-grandson for his fifth birthday. Words cease to be weapons, or challenges, or clues, but become instead a form of solace, a litany of love and tenderness. As Vivian is lulled into fitful sleep, her professor leans closer. Moving seamlessly from nursery chant to Shakespeare, she whispers to her dying student the same soft words with which Horatio bids farewell to his friend, a poisoned Hamlet: 'And flights of angels sing thee to thy rest.'

Wit was both a warning and a plea. It cautioned us against browbeating our future patients while beseeching us to recognise the healing potential of small acts of kindness. But empathy – the ability to understand and identify with the feelings of another – was under assault from day one of medical school. With biochemistry and anatomy filling our days, one way or another, people were reduced – either to chemical interactions or to corpses on slabs. In this first, most formative year of medical school, the dead, not the living, took centre stage.

I strongly suspected from the outset that the real point of human dissection was to kickstart the process of detachment. In a contemporary culture that likes to keep its dead behind closed doors, once you have crossed the line into a life steeped in body parts – the stench of refrigerated flesh slowly rotting in formaldehyde never quite leaving your clothes – there is no going back. You have seen and sliced and smelt too much. We were a cohort of students who needed first to be dehumanised, then rebuilt as doctors.

The anatomy room was our site of metamorphosis. I was filled with trepidation before crossing its threshold. Dad had told me that in his day the dissection room was a place from which medical students used to commandeer body parts for laughs. Back then, in the 1960s, after a long day flaying human sinew, nerve and skin, they liked to unwind by terrorising unsuspecting punters with pub pranks involving human hands and eyeballs, purloined when the anatomists' backs were turned.

'You know the kind of thing, Rachel,' he told me. 'You'd get someone to shake hands with you but offer them the one you'd dissected earlier. They'd drop their pint in horror when it came away in their palm.'

'Honestly, Dad, I *don't* know. I mean, I can't begin to imagine you doing that. It's completely repulsive.'

It was also, if I were honest, completely unnerving. If doctors were the kind of people who, even as students, found human dismemberment hilarious, then was I really cut out for medicine? Or, had Dad once instinctively recoiled like me, yet emerged from his time among the silver-slabbed dead with his memory erased of the qualms he had once felt upon taking a scalpel to their cold, embalmed flesh?

For all my misgivings, when I entered the dissection room myself for the very first time the smell of concentrated formaldehyde was oddly familiar. It was, I realised, a scent I had encountered before as a child: whenever I collected too many owl pellets to dissect all at once, I preserved some in small jars, supplied by Dad, ready to delve into after another week at school. Maybe this would not be too bad, I thought hopefully.

A preserved body, I discovered, is so stiff and cold from its refrigerated store that it no more feels like flesh than a waxwork. As long as I did not look too closely at the face, I could pretend what I was doing – coaxing away human hide with my blade – was vaguely normal. Any feelings of revulsion were surprisingly short-lived and, better yet, swiftly superseded by the genuine delight of learning through cutting. For the next year, six of us spent two mornings a week gloved and gowned, stooped over the corpse of a man in his eighties whom we steadily whittled away to bare bones, having politely christened him 'Henry'.

'Oh my God, look at this!' Will exclaimed one day. We had incised Henry's chest from top to bottom, then peeled back the skin to expose his ribcage. After crunching his way through the ribs with metal cutters, Will had exposed Henry's lungs to the light, and their appearance shocked us all. 'Look at them! How many pack years has he put behind him?' We gawped at lungs so blackened and scarred they looked like they'd been attacked with a blowtorch. One 'pack year' was twenty cigarettes a day, 365 days a year. Henry had surely smoked untipped Woodbines for decades. Here, before our incredulous eyes, was the cumulative effect of half a million cigarettes, a core of rotting tar in his chest, almost certainly the cause of his demise.

Eagerly, we burrowed and rummaged for tumour. 'There's bound to be a cancer in here, there must be,' I muttered, gouging deeper with my scalpel. Sure enough, a knobbly, craggy, malignant mass lurked within one lung field.

'Wow,' said Will. 'That is . . . impressively disgusting.'

The dry textbook descriptions of 'tobacco smoker's lung' had just leapt off the page, reeking of formaldehyde, and its visceral reality – how disease actually looked, felt and smelt in our hands – was unforgettable. For the rest of the day, alongside the lingering trace of preservatives, I wore an unshakeable grin. This five-year project of transformation into a doctor – I was loving it.

I was fortunate enough to be part of a generation of doctors whose first hands-on encounters with the human bodies we dissected were infused with respect, not ribaldry. Our anatomy professor demanded something close to reverence. He expected us to recognise, and to be humbled by, the last act of generosity from the nameless souls who, in the name of helping others, had bequeathed their bodies to our hesitant blades. Following his lead, we took our scalpels' defacements seriously.

What had not changed, however, since my father's day was the peculiar act of doublethink required for young men and women, most of them still teenagers, to cluster, scalpels poised, around a slowly decomposing corpse while loudly pretending that carving up dead human flesh was a perfectly anodyne use of Tuesday and Thursday mornings. Our experience of dissection may have been respectful, it may have had the vital aim of rendering us fluent in human anatomy, but it could not, in any sense of the term, have been described as normal. This was an act of violation – the mutilation of the dead, their physical defilement – that tugged at our species' darkest taboos, and yet at no point was this ever discussed openly.

In failing to acknowledge the enormity of what occurred behind the dissection room doors, our tutors unwittingly taught us something profound. That around the dead swirled unspeakable secrets. That, as fledgling doctors-to-be, our new role required us to stifle, not voice, our feelings and instincts. That any emotions provoked were illegitimate and gauche. That we had to ignore and deny them. That if, instead, we admitted our vulnerabilities when up close with death, we were something of an embarrassment to medicine.

Many of us, I suspect, clung with silent gratitude to the task of naming each tiny scrap of the human form. In the gargantuan effort of committing to memory several thousand Latin labels for every muscle, nerve and bone, came the relief of intellectual detachment. We could keep our weakness under wraps.

There is nothing quite like flirting with death to inspire unguarded living. Immediately before starting medical school I began dating my future husband. On 20 March 2003, the first day of the Iraq War, the sum total of my acquaintance with Dave had been one blind date a year earlier, a date so embarrassing, so excruciatingly awkward, the details must remain forever classified. And yet, ever since that catastrophic evening, I had been unable to suppress the unnerving thought that out of all the men who had ever lived, this one, the catastrophe, was the only one for me. Clearly, a normal person would have done something about this, but I was English, so would have rather roasted my eyeballs. A year had elapsed, and all I had done was sigh wistfully.

Then, three days after the Iraq War began, a Royal Air Force fast jet, a Tornado GR4, was accidentally shot down by an American missile as it returned from a bombing raid over Baghdad. Both pilot and navigator were killed instantly, and the British public swiftly learned a new vocabulary – 'blue-on-blue' and 'fratricide' – to denote not Cain-and-Abel-style brotherly slaughter but military comrades killing their own in error.

Amid the soaring death toll in Iraq – we all knew what the Pentagon's 'shock and awe' tactics meant for the civilians upon whom the bombs rained down – the loss of two unnamed British airmen should not have haunted me. But Dave, the man I had not set eyes on for a year yet somehow never stopped longing for, was himself a Royal Air Force fighter pilot. For all I knew, he had been flying that jet. I lay awake at night aching to know whether he were still alive, while cursing myself for being bashful, not gutsy, never finding out what he might have meant to me.

The next day I received an email from an address I did not recognise. From a military tent in a scorched Saudi desert, my fighter pilot, shocked by the death of his comrades, had thrown caution to the wind and decided to contact me. Liberated by distance and the precariousness of life, we started writing to each other with gleeful abandon, the kind of candour you lose with your childhood. Aside from the topics the military censors could object to, everything and nothing was covered with impunity. Life, death, dreams, trivia, all that we hoped for from the future, should we be so lucky to be granted one.

By the time Dave returned from Iraq, I already knew I wanted to marry him. In an attempt to downplay my feelings, I arranged our second date in an East London curry house lined with maroon velour wallpaper – the least romantic, lowest-stakes encounter possible. To no avail. When I started pouring water over the tablecloth – I had been aiming for his glass, but had been distracted by his cheekbones – I knew I was hopelessly, horribly smitten. Later that week, as I held a human heart – Henry's heart – in my hands, in my head I was composing bad love poetry.

For all the early focus on corpses, death was conspicuous by its absence from the student curriculum. Nowhere at my medical school, even in the scant hours dedicated to honing our communication skills with patients, was there open discussion of the fears in which dying is so often steeped. It was perfectly clear that, just as Vivian Bearing used her prodigious intellect to deflect her mortal fears, so too were many of the doctors who taught us sidestepping the matter of death themselves.

In their case, the shield of choice was actions, not words. So long as those tutoring tomorrow's doctors focused strictly on doing – the diagnosing, the treating, the saving, the controlling – then dying could safely be downplayed, even ignored. Yet death, of course, was all around us. The hospital was full of it. Troops of elephants were stampeding through every ward.

This could lead to some painful moments. Once, as a student, I was attached to a medical team who admitted a patient with severe chest pain and breathlessness, and an underlying diagnosis of cancer of the kidney.

Timothy Bradbrooke was a dignified former professor of linguistics. Now in his seventies, he still wielded words with magnificent precision, much like Vivian Bearing herself. Since malignancy makes the blood more prone to clotting, the medics suspected he had developed a pulmonary embolism, a clot in his lung. A scan appeared to confirm the finding until a second, more senior radiologist took a look. As expert opinions bounced back and forth, Professor Bradbrooke languished with his wife behind curtains in the emergency department, wondering what was taking so long. Eventually, a consensus was reached, and my consultant set off to explain the diagnosis, along with several other doctors and five or six medical students in tow.

We were quite a pack. Around ten of us loomed above the Bradbrookes like stethoscoped harbingers of doom. Undeterred, the consultant began his explanation. 'Well, Professor Bradbrooke, would you like the good news or the bad news?' This was a rhetorical question. Without missing a beat, he continued, 'The good news is, you don't have a pulmonary embolism. The bad news, though, is that what we thought was a blood clot is, in fact, cancer. The tumour in your kidney has spread up the vena cava and seeded in your heart. So that opacity on your scan is actually cancer. Highly unusual. Never seen it myself before.'

I was watching Professor Bradbrooke closely. He blanched. The import of the words stripped his face of its poise and, for a moment, I saw fear surge. Suddenly, there was insufficient space inside the cubicle to breathe. We, the medics, were blotting out all the air.

'W-what do you mean, cancer in the heart?' his wife asked.

'It's called a metastasis. Distant spread,' answered the consultant, as though Mrs Bradbrooke were seeking etymological clarity.

The questions, clearly, were more existential. How can my husband have cancer in his heart? If the cancer is there – in *there*, of all places – is he dying? Is this it? Am I losing him? I could have been wrong. But I had glimpsed it in her husband's eyes as well – the shock of confronting your own death, uncloaked and raw.

Every word spoken from this point on might just as well have been scattered like dust on the wind. Nothing held. The consultant was droning about referrals, further scans, a transfer to the oncology ward, but the Bradbrookes, holding hands, were stupefied.

If ever there was a time for kindness, this was it. Fear swamped the little cubicle. Husband and wife stared wide-eyed. I waited for a human connection between doctor and patient, for the consultant to offer a word, a hand, anything to signify to this man at his moment of mortal reckoning that he was not being cast aside.

There was nothing. Either the consultant was oblivious of the devastation he had just unleashed, or else he was running away from it. We swept onwards, following his lead, another twenty or more patients waiting to be seen on the round. One of us should have gone back. *I* should have gone back. Instead, we closed the curtains like a veil on the elderly woman who clung on, with all her might, to the man with the cancer in his heart.

The process of being wrenched, as medical students, ever further from normal social conventions – while being taught to suppress our emotional response to mortality – unfolded first with dead bodies, and next with live ones. Dave, my now husband-to-be, winced in disbelief at some of the stories I brought home with me. Early on, as an inexperienced medical student, I was instructed by a ward doctor to take blood from an inpatient. Eager to oblige, hungry to prove my competence, I gathered my tourniquet and needles and set off to find the patient.

I was drawn up short. The man from whom I had been told to take blood almost glowed from his bed, such was the depth of his jaundice. The contours of his face wore no softening of flesh, his eyes were too small for their sockets. I was looking at a skull wrapped in yellow-tinted clingfilm. My instinct, suppressed, was to recoil. Here was a man evidently so close to death that his grasp on life seemed absurd, outlandish. How could he still be alive? I could not understand what possible extra facts a tubeful of blood could add to the situation.

I hovered uncertainly at the nurses' station, scared, if I was honest, to approach him. Feeling out of my depth, I bought myself some time by leafing through his medical notes. Pancreatic cancer, run rampant. Typically, a furious, aggressive disease. No wonder the man looked so haunted. Nervously, as though his proximity to dying could somehow infect me, I approached the bedside. What I was doing felt wrong, yet I buried my reticence, just as medical school had taught me.

'Hello, Mr Smith,' I said, with inappropriate breeziness. 'My name is Rachel, and I'm a medical student. I've been asked to take some blood. It should only take a moment.'

I fear I did not, proactively, ask his permission for the blood-taking. And that I chose to take as consent the way he stared mutely into my eyes, because I did not want to fail the doctor who had sent me there. Proceeding did not simply feel wrong, I *knew* it was wrong, but I went ahead anyway, telling myself it was necessary as I tightened my tourniquet on bone.

Suddenly, he grimaced, teeth bared. 'Why won't you all just stop torturing me?' he muttered weakly. 'Why can't you just fuck off and leave me alone to die?'

Horrified, I saw myself through his eyes. In following orders, against my better judgement, I was indeed inflicting a tiny act of torture – the sting of my needle as pointless as it was callous. Mortified, apologising, I scuttled away, returning empty-handed to my team.

'I'm sorry. He doesn't want anyone to take blood any more,' I told the doctor.

'Oh. Well – yeah – fair enough, I guess. It's not like the results are going to change anything, the state he's in,' said my senior. It was all I could do not to retort in fury, 'Well, why the hell couldn't you have figured that out before telling me to go and stab him?'

The fact was, my rage was really directed at myself. My instincts, my feelings, had been right, but still I had continued to act wrongly. I may have convinced myself the proper doctors knew better than me, that there was a reason for the blood-taking beyond my understanding, but my reluctant obedience had just trumped my human decency. I felt I might be joining a club I did not want to be a part of.

On one level, I recognised that inadvertent cruelty was an inevitable risk in a profession whose essential requirement is the tempering of empathy with detachment. We might have chosen medicine because we wanted to help people, but doctors could not and should not allow their compassion free rein. If an oncologist, for example, permitted herself truly to share the pain of her twenty-eight-year-old patient dying of breast cancer, inconsolable at leaving her children, then how could she compute the treatment permutations most likely to maximise the quality of her patient's remaining life? How would she do her job?

No one, I knew, deserved a doctor weeping at their bedside when hard medical expertise was what would help them. The challenge, then, for every doctor was to acquire sufficient detachment to be useful, while maintaining one's essential humanity. But, as students, no one ever discussed this with us. Indeed, doctors did not seem to acknowledge the emotional toll of their work at all, affecting, instead, to take it blithely in their stride.

*

My first two years of medical school were a whirlwind of biochemistry, anatomy, physiology and pathology. I forgot all about Vivian Bearing. My aim, like everybody else's, was excelling in exams, and that required precision and certainty, not mumbo-jumbo metaphysics. Indeed, the multiple choice tests to which we were constantly subjected required us not only to select the right answer, but also to grade with a 1, 2 or 3 how confident we were that we were right, with 3 conveying either total faith in your answer or your willingness to take a gamble. Over-confidence incurred a penalty, but if you selected a '3' and were correct, you received bonus marks for audacity. It was therefore possible to earn a score of 150 per cent on every exam, 50 per cent better than perfect. Needless to say, nothing less satisfied me.

Even while obediently jumping through these hoops, I was aware that this method of marking inculcated attitude as well as knowledge. It seemed my university not only wanted its medics erudite, we had to be risk-takers as well. Apparently, there was no place for doubt in medicine: hesitate and you shall be chastised.

But over-confidence has its drawbacks. Arrogance and reflective practice do not go hand in hand. Occasionally, while trotting obediently behind a hospital consultant, I saw direct evidence that the exploitative relationship between doctor and patient depicted so vividly in *Wit* had not entirely vanished. Once, on a student attachment in neurology, eight of us assembled before an eminent professor to begin our weekly bedside teaching session.

'Right,' Professor Melrose announced dramatically. 'I have a treat for you this morning. You will be very lucky if you ever see anything like this again.' I felt a stab of unease in the pit of my stomach. I had a feeling I knew what was coming. 'Follow me, boys and girls! Bed 3A.'

With a flourish of his wrist, he swept down the corridor, his gaggle of students scuttling after him. I had only a moment in which to make a decision. I knew exactly who lay in Bed 3A, and exactly why it was out of the question that the nine of us should descend upon her.

Bed 3A contained Maureen Gibson, a woman in her early sixties. I had met her when she had first arrived in the emergency department, and made a point of catching up with her daily ever since. For some months, Maureen had been vaguely aware of feeling weaker than usual. In order to lift herself out of her armchair she found she needed to grip on to the sides with both hands. Soon, her arms as well as legs seemed sapped of strength. Reaching up into a kitchen cupboard to take down a tin of soup became an exercise in trying to ignore her new-found frailty. Eventually, one morning, as she tried to answer the telephone, the receiver slipped from her feeble grasp. As it lay out of reach on the carpet, her fear of not knowing what was happening to her body finally outstripped that of learning the answer. She asked her husband to drive her to hospital.

Behind a flimsy curtain, under green-tinged lights, I met Maureen with a neurology registrar. The clamour, moaning, clattering and bleeping of an A&E in full swing was only a sliver of polyester away. The fear in Maureen's eyes belied her defiant cheer.

'I'm wondering if this could just be a vitamin deficiency?' she asked, hopefully. 'My diet's been pretty rubbish lately. Or maybe it's just down to stress at work recently?'

I could see she did not believe a word of it.

'That's right,' interjected her husband, hastily. 'She's been working far too hard. Honestly, she hasn't had a break for months. That's going to have an impact, isn't it?'

Gently, respectfully, the neurologist first took Maureen's history, then carefully examined her body. His compassion astounded me. As expected, Maureen's limbs were exceptionally weak. More surprising were her reflexes. Most people have an impressive knee jerk. Tap the tendon beneath the kneecap with a patella hammer, and the shin swings upwards, signalling that muscles and nerves are working as they should. Other reflexes are harder to elicit, some requiring great skill from the doctor attempting to assess their briskness. But Maureen's whole body was overrun with florid twitching. Tap almost any part of her, however lightly, and it would jerk involuntarily. Even a fingertip to her chin caused her jaw to jerk open in a spasm. I struggled to keep my face serene, a blank canvas. I had never seen anything like it.

The neurologist quietly explained that to get to the bottom of the symptoms, Maureen would need to be admitted to our ward for further investigation. After we left her bedside, he grilled me. 'What's the diagnosis, Rachel? What's the one thing you want to rule out?' Maureen's neurological findings fitted one particular dread diagnosis, that of motor neurone disease. A progressive and ultimately fatal disease, MND is caused by gradual degeneration of a type of nerve, the motor neurones, in the brain and spinal cord. There is no cure.

Over the coming days, the overwhelming likelihood of this bleak diagnosis was discussed in many conversations with Maureen. The rapidity of her decline terrified her. Daily, it seemed, she could feel herself weakening. The prospect of becoming steadily imprisoned inside a failing body – first wheelchair-bound, then unable to feed and, finally, even to breathe unaided – was almost unbearably frightening.

I took to arriving half an hour early on the ward when I could in order to visit Maureen. As a medical student, I had the luxury of time in which to do so. Sometimes we simply sat in silence, her hand clasped in mine, tears flowing. On better days, we chatted. I learned all about the day she first set eyes on her husband, and how much her grandson loved stamping through puddles.

Word quickly spread through the hospital that there was an MND patient on Neurology with clinical signs so startlingly severe you might only see them once in your career. A steady stream of students and doctors began to flock to Maureen's bedside. Patiently, she endured the poking and prodding over and over again. But there are limits. The disease that had made her a medical curio was also, steadily, incarcerating her. The crowds she drew only served to underline how unusual, and exceptionally unpleasant, her fate was.

There is only so much gawping a person can take. For Maureen, the morning of the professorial teaching round was crunch point. Earlier, she had told me through her tears that she could not face anyone wanting to examine her today. As Professor Melrose strode towards her bedside, I called out to him from behind.

'Excuse me, Prof. Melrose. Please stop. We can't see this patient.'

He turned to face me, eyes flashing with anger. 'And who, exactly, are you?' he barked.

I moved closer, not wanting to be overheard, and murmured diffidently, 'I know this patient. I was there when she was admitted. She was crying this morning and she doesn't want any students.'

'I beg your pardon? I'll be the judge of that,' he retorted, and set off again towards Bay 3.

'No,' I blurted, louder.

He swung back towards me, glowering. My fellow students looked on. Professor Melrose had a daunting reputation for tearing strips off his juniors, frequently reducing them to tears. I was torn between standing my ground and shrivelling up before him. It helped being a decade older than my peers.

Silence. I held his stare. Then, with the briefest of nods in my direction, he stalked off to find another patient.

'Well, Rach, I hope to Christ you don't get him as your examiner at the end of this rotation,' someone muttered.

'The sooner he retires the better,' I whispered in reply.

A few weeks later, Dad called me. 'So, how did the exam go?'

That morning, each of us had examined a patient before the hawkish eyes of a consultant neurologist. Inevitably, I had been assigned Professor Melrose. The case was impossibly hard. My patient's curious combination of malfunctioning eye movements occurred in a condition so rare, most textbooks neglected to mention it. As I struggled to make sense of the neuroanatomical signs I had elicited, I refused on principle to flinch from Melrose's glare. To my surprise, as the bell rang for me to move on to the next patient, his expression momentarily softened.

'The woman with MND, Rachel,' he muttered. 'You were right to insist we left her alone. Thank you.'

I told Dad what had happened. It seemed to matter more than the latest academic hoop. 'I think,' Dad mused, reflecting back on his decades of doctoring, 'that you can end up immune to other people's pain precisely because you started out with compassion. You don't want to turn cold, but it hurts too much not to be. You can't keep on going otherwise.'

I thought of what Melrose's daily clinics entailed. As an expert in movement disorders, he endured the experience, day in, day out, of revealing to new patients one of an array of dreadful diagnoses. Parkinson's disease, progressive supranuclear palsy, corticobasal degeneration, multiple system atrophy. Some of the most remorseless, incurable, vicious diseases whose names and bleakness he inflicted on others, over and over again. Could I really say with conviction that I would survive decades of dropping bombshells that shattered my patients' lives with my warmth and humanity intact? Could any of us, with confidence, claim that?

4

Ghost Owl

Illness is the night side of life, a more onerous citizenship.
Everyone who is born holds dual citizenship, in the kingdom of
the well and in the kingdom of the sick. Although we all prefer to
use the good passport, sooner or later each of us is obliged, at least
for a spell, to identify ourselves as citizens of that other place.

Susan Sontag, *Illness as Metaphor*

I did not expect to mimic Vivian Bearing so soon after watching her fictional fate. But agape I lay, defenceless in stirrups, eyes fixed on the silver blades of the fan that was singularly failing to deflect from my face the smell of my own burning body. A man, a gynaecologist, was at work between my legs. I had never longed more strongly to slip my skin, to be disembodied. Anything, but anything to be shot of this posture and these restraints around my ankles.

This was not, in my case, an indignity of cancer. No one had even mentioned that word. This was nothing, a trifle, compared to other patients' experiences – and I knew this better than most. I had taken the call that had led me to this room, this couch, mid-way through my medical school gynaecology attachment. In my hospital, I had discovered, the cutting, ablating, paring and splicing of women's bodies was primarily the handicraft of men. One of the male gynaecologists had presented a recent cohort of students with a handwritten, photocopied guide he had entitled 'Gynaecology at your fingertips'. Behind his back, the nurses called him Goldfinger, whether in reference to his Ferrari or his skill in certain aspects of his practice I was never entirely certain.

Some of the women who populated the gynaecology ward had endured surgeries so extreme they warranted their own macabre vocabulary. An 'exenteration', I learned in my first week – from the Latin *enteron*, meaning 'intestine', and *ex*, meaning 'out of' – referred to the complete disembowelment of a body cavity. Female pelvic exenteration entailed the surgical removal of the bladder, urethra, rectum, anus, vagina, cervix, uterus and ovaries. Small wonder these women appeared eerily impassive, lying still as statues beneath white hospital cotton, as though shrouded to protect us from what their bodies had so violently become. I wanted to sit and talk and listen, to reach the mothers and sisters beneath the drains and tubes, but the scale of the mutilation scared me. I could not bear to imagine bodies scraped this bare, excavated so thoroughly.

At night, I found myself reading medical history. So-called heroic surgery, inspired by the efforts of surgeons during the Second World War, had intoxicated the profession in the post-war era. Alexander Brunschwig, the American surgeon who invented total pelvic exenteration, extolled the virtues of radical excision to cure his patients of gynaecological cancer.

Evidence for his methods was scant, but the *British Medical Journal*, reviewing one of his books in 1948, commented enthusiastically: 'After perusing the book everyone will agree that he is a bold, skilful, courageous and optimistic surgeon.' I couldn't help but feel that for Mr Brunschwig, the female body was a territory to conquer and subjugate, and that the courage lay in those being surgically plundered. Remarkably, the *BMJ* continued: 'The author does not allow the idea of prognosis to affect his definition of "operable". He defines an operable neoplasm as "one that can be excised regardless of where or how much spread has developed".' In other words, so long as Brunschwig felt the patient would not actually expire upon the table, then their body was fair game and radical surgery worth pursuing. Thirty-four of the hundred patients described in the book died during or immediately after surgery. Heroism was bloody work.

As I sat in a lecture about gynaecological cancers, my GP had called to reveal the results of my recent cervical smear test. For a moment I thought she was simply being thoughtful, making a special effort to speak directly to a fellow female professional. Then: 'It's nothing to worry about, Rachel, but the test has come back as positive.'

Of course. Doctors do not call their patients to impart run-of-the-mill good news. I endeavoured to sound relaxed and knowledgeable. 'Oh . . . I see. Well, thanks for calling. I expect it's CIN 1, isn't it?'

'Actually, no. It's CIN 3.' She paused. 'So, I'll refer you to the colposcopy clinic. They'll probably want to see you within the week.'

'Ah, OK.' The pause was now mine. 'Well, that's very kind

of you to let me know. Thank you,' I said breezily, determined to avoid sounding neurotic. Then, I crept out of the back of the lecture hall to where the hospital assembled its bodily waste bins, knowing that even the most hardened smokers steered clear of spots as unsavoury as this one. I stood very still and tried not to panic, feeling weak and small.

CIN, cervical intraepithelial neoplasia, is pronounced 'sin' and carries, in some minds, vaguely licentious connotations. These deformed, misshapen cells – which, if left untreated, can transform into cancer – are strongly associated with a sexually transmitted infection, human papilloma virus. Only very rarely will a woman who is sexually inactive develop cervical cancer. 'Good girls', in short, are protected, while 'bad girls' put themselves at risk. All of this rushed over me, snatching the air from my lungs. Somehow, I felt judged, as well as imperilled. What had I done wrong? Was this my fault? Above all, the terrible thought that I might share the fate of the shrouded women and be forced to face the men whose scalpels dealt in evisceration.

CIN came in three degrees of severity. My kind was the worst, requiring total excision. Only when – if – the margins came back clear would I know I had not developed cancer. Colposcopy – inspection of the cervix under a microscope – would in my case be followed by a 'loop excision' of the affected area. A cheese wire, in essence, incandescent with electrical current, would slice away the edge of my cervix along with, in theory, any trace of malignancy. The procedure, if unpleasant, required only gritted teeth and a strong stomach. It was the fear of invasion that undid me. I tried to banish all thoughts of a future in freefall, children I would never bear, a husband I would never grow old with, the years of beautiful, glorious life shrinking down to a vista of pain and drains and scars, and the bitterness of everything being cancerous.

On returning home that evening, I hid my fear from Dave – because what possible benefit could come from infecting him? Medical school had already taught me that the facts one chose to omit carried at least as much weight as those uttered. So, I mentioned only an abnormal smear, the need for a second test, its minor nature. No need for terms like 'neoplasia' that might invite him to share my catastrophising.

'Are you worried?' he asked, searching my face for the answer.

'No, not at all,' I smiled back at him. 'The statistics are totally in my favour. It's going to be fine.'

A few days later, I arrived at the colposcopy clinic. I had kept my NHS ID card round my neck like a forlorn plastic amulet, as if a name badge could somehow ward off the transition from professional to patient, with all the loss of power – the diminishment – that entailed. I knew it was the condition, not the doctors, that had conferred my newfound vulnerability, yet still I found myself wanting to blame the stethoscoped messengers.

The gynaecologist, a professor, was close to retirement. Thousands of women like me had walked through his door, brave faces on, defiance disguising nothing. He smiled, an expression of genuine warmth that instantly cut through my defensiveness. 'I'd like to suggest, if I may, Rachel, that I treat you not as a medical student but simply as a patient. It doesn't really matter how much someone knows or doesn't know about a condition. The facts are not the same as the experience. Are you happy with that?' he asked.

Happy was stretching it, but the relief, in those moments, was overwhelming. He was kind, it was clear, and what his patients felt mattered to him. Even as I stripped off my underwear, for the first time since the phone call I felt safe again.

Diathermy, in abstract, has an irresistible elegance. Using electricity to heat metal creates surgical tools that sculpt and sear simultaneously. Flesh is sealed as it is cut, minimising blood loss beautifully. The reality – your own charred flesh, acrid in your nostrils – is harder to appreciate. I gripped the hand of the nurse like my life depended on it, and when my legs started to tremble, and she told me I was being brave, I wanted to hug her with gratitude. How had nobody taught me through my years of medical school the sheer power of these small acts of kindness, and of simple human touch to transcend primal fear?

The margins, it transpired, were clear. I had been granted a reprieve. But this time, unlike my previous brushes with mortality, I vowed never to dismiss the experience. The fear I had felt, the surge of blind panic, this was how it had begun for every woman on my ward. My brush with cancer, however fleeting, had revealed a glimpse of the abyss. I had acquired something vital: a means to empathise more fully with my patients, an ability I never knew I lacked.

There was more. That night, lying in bed with Dave, the close encounter with cancer still lingering like formaldehyde, we talked about the precariousness of life. Everything we had taken for granted – our careers, a family, the future fat with promise – had been planned in blithe denial of our own fragility. 'But what else can you do?' mused Dave. 'All you can do is choose life.'

I knew he was right. The only alternative to unguarded living – to hurling yourself hopefully into an unknown future – was a pinched, pale, drab existence in which nothing could be lost, since nothing had been invested of your human heart. And who would want to live like that?

'Maybe,' I speculated sleepily, 'you only *really* appreciate the joy of being alive when you accept that all of it, every single one of your experiences, is destined to be lost. *That's* when you savour it. Maybe death makes us love life.'

Dave raised a sceptical eyebrow. 'I've no idea about that, but I do have an excellent suggestion.' He smiled and leaned closer. 'Let's start a family.'

'Ooh, this is a good one for you, Rach. Have you ever been taught how to do a breast exam?' a fresh-faced man in scrubs asked me.

'No,' I answered eagerly, 'but I'd love to learn.'

We were talking in Minors, the section of the emergency department where patients who are well enough to walk into hospital are directed. Across the way, in Majors, lay the more seriously unwell who are rushed to our care by ambulance. Ed, the doctor in charge of Minors that day, had taken me under his wing. As a medical student I was dead space, an inconvenience, acutely aware of my ability to get under the feet of the proper doctors and nurses. At six foot four, with a rugby player's body and outsized personality to match, Ed dominated the department. His favourite form of emergency medicine was being scrambled on to an air ambulance and helicoptered into bedlam to rescue the smashed and crushed and maimed from chaos. Motorway pile-ups, major fires and explosions – adrenalin-charged Action Man stuff.

In the humdrum cubicles of Minors, patients were seen in strict arrival order, and the next on the list, a twenty-year-old woman named Fabiana, had an unusual reason for attending. 'Who comes to A&E for a breast lump?' Ed speculated. 'It doesn't make sense. Maybe she's a student and doesn't have a GP or something.'

I was intrigued. Inside her cubicle, barely hidden from view by the flimsy polyester curtain, Fabiana perched rigidly on the edge of her chair, hands clenched tight into fists. She looked like one wrong word might cause her to bolt. Ed, normally exuberant to the point of boisterousness, now spoke quietly, gently, as though trying to pacify a cornered animal, while her eyes darted anxiously between us. Gradually, he coaxed out a story of sorts. I knew queues of patients were overwhelming the department, yet he conveyed the erroneous impression of having all the time in the world.

Fabiana's Spanish accent was hard to understand, but eventually we gleaned that she had come to the UK for six months to learn English. She did, in fact, have a GP, but they had already examined her and concluded no lump was present. The GP, like Ed, had taken a detailed history. Fabiana had no family history of breast cancer, or any other risk factors. This trip to A&E was, in essence, a peculiar attempt to obtain a second opinion. Seemingly in perfect, almost lustrous health, she had waited five hours to see us.

Ed asked permission to examine her himself, though suggesting she might prefer to see a female doctor. She shook her head. She wanted it over with. Unbuttoning her blouse, she seemed to shrink in size, visibly flinching as Ed approached. Unclothed, she looked more child than adult, thin and infinitely fragile. With one glance, Ed signalled to me that there was no question of teaching – and I loved him for it. Myself, I longed to wrap

her in blankets for protection. Respectfully, methodically –
thoroughness was essential – he palpated each breast in turn,
probing deep into each armpit, searching every cranny where
cancer can lurk undiscovered. Fabiana stared up at the ceiling,
biting her lip for distraction. I noticed her mobile phone on the
desk beside her, decorated with stickers of koalas and Pikachu.

It was over. Ed waited until she was fully clothed, then
revealed what he assumed was good news, that he had found
nothing. Her eyes fell to the floor. I saw tears begin to glint in
their corners. Ed watched carefully as she gathered her phone
and pulled on her jacket. This was the moment to move on, get
cracking with seeing the next patient. Instead, just as she was
about to walk out, he reached a hand towards her.

'Fabiana, please wait. I think there is a reason you came to
see us today, something you're finding it hard to tell us.'

She hesitated, hand on the curtain.

'It's OK,' he told her. 'Perhaps, if you feel you can tell us,
we can help you?'

Her face began to crumple. She sat back down, tears flowing.
'My sister,' she sobbed. 'My sister.'

In fits and starts, the story emerged. At only twenty-five,
Fabiana's older sister was in a Spanish hospital receiving
chemotherapy for metastatic breast cancer. Genetic testing had
revealed an underlying mutation, BRCA1, that dramatically
increases the risk of developing the disease, and Fabiana was at
significant risk of having also inherited it. Her sister's cancer
was virulent, unstoppable, the chemotherapy merely an attempt
to eke out a little more time, a palliative intervention.

'Did you mention this to your GP?' asked Ed.

Fabiana shook her head. She had felt unable to do so.

The family history of BRCA1 changed everything. For all the reassurance of a normal examination, the odds were suddenly skewed towards cancer. But a visit to the hospital's one-stop breast lump clinic for a scan and assessment by an oncologist was not simply prudent. Here was a girl, scarcely a woman, who was looking on as cancer, in relentless bites, claimed her sister's life, and who was terrified she shared the same fate. Even if all a scan achieved was reassurance, denying her that chance would have been inhuman.

We made some calls, squeezed her into a clinic, and watched her disappear down the corridor. Then, on an impulse, she turned and rushed back towards Ed. Still crying, she flung her arms around him. 'Thank you, doctor. Thank you.'

What I learned that day was immeasurably more important than the manual mechanics of conducting a breast examination. The sensitivity of this burly, brawny bull of a man, his skill at helping a vulnerable young woman feel able to trust him. Above all, his understanding of why, amid the intensity and constraints of A&E, unravelling the human crisis within this particular cubicle had been so very vital. I stored away his example of tact and compassion, knowing I would draw on it in years to come, as I drew so often on my father's. Of one thing I was certain. Fabiana would forget him no sooner than I would.

If I could prescribe anything at medical school, it would be a decent dose of temporary illness, one for every future doctor. Something sufficiently grave to stoke genuine fear, involving at least a couple of distasteful procedures, the mere thought of which would make the students squirm. Perhaps a colonoscopy apiece, alongside a diagnosis that spelt potential catastrophe. Otherwise, how can they truly understand what it is that a patient submits to, the scale of doctors' demands upon the unwell?

It is fair to say that I am not a person who likes instruction, least of all under duress. Yet, as a patient, I am meekness personified. Turn this way, look up to the ceiling, straighten your arm, open your legs, just pop up on this couch. Patients oblige, comply, obey; they cannot risk dissent when so much power is concentrated in medical hands. There is, incidentally, a special place in hell reserved for doctors who ask people to 'pop'. Neither adults nor children 'pop' their clothes off, women do not 'pop' their cherries (or anything else, for that matter) and nothing, but nothing, is benign about medical couches, no matter how jovially a doctor pretends that 'popping' up on them is normal. You might slink or creep or tiptoe towards that shiny, plastic, ominous cheapness, steeling yourself to surrender your body, but never do you jauntily spring there.

Every time I encountered a doctor with Ed's heart and kindness – and there were so many throughout my training – I glimpsed a little more of what mattered in medicine. But it was seeing things, if briefly, from the other side – the harsh and alien realm of the unwell – that really opened my eyes. The surge of fear at the thought of a possible cancer growing unseen inside you, the fight not to cry as your cervix burns, your identity shrinking into the slip of plastic around your wrist, your consternation at being barcoded like a tin of beans in Tesco.

And then there are the lessons about sheer, desperate impotence that no one can teach you like a person you love, someone you would do anything not to lose – someone who, even as they make your life brighter, must face their own being cut down.

*

They say a medical degree requires committing three million facts to memory. When I walked into my first end-of-year exams, I was brittle with sleeplessness, having fretted away the night before. On one level, I knew there was no doubt I would pass – this twitchiness was born out of wanting to excel – but still, it all seemed so terribly important. Head down, focus total, three hours swept by while I poured out my brain on to the paper. Someone was escorted from the examination hall sobbing. The collective scratching of three hundred pens sounded like a meerkat invasion.

Several hundred miles away, in a small district hospital, a woman had just arrived by ambulance. Pat, Dave's mother, was critically ill. Shocked, frightened, overwhelmed with septicaemia, an infection running rampant through her blood. The first I knew of the crisis was when I turned on my phone. Twelve missed calls, all from Dave. While I'd been regurgitating reams of medical facts – a vanity exercise, aiming for prizes – he had tried and tried to reach me. My stomach lurched. Even as I called him, I knew the news would be dreadful.

'Hey. It's me. Darling, what's happened?'

From far away – the realm of lost loved ones – he answered. Clipped, terse, military precision. 'It's Mum. She's in hospital. I'm on my way there.' I gleaned scraps of information, incomplete and confusing. All he had really understood from his father was that he had to get there, and now.

That night, on his return from the hospital, we spoke again, this time at length. The critical fact, the one that knocked the rest away, was that Pat was so unwell her chances of surviving her septicaemia were, at most, fifty-fifty. Worse, scans had revealed a devastating finding. Cancer, widely spread, invading everywhere. So even if she made it through the next few days, her future still hung in the balance.

'I can come up tomorrow. I'll resit the exams. I'll be there by lunchtime,' I told him.

'No, don't be silly. Get your exams out of the way. Come when they're over.'

I could hardly stand the strain in Dave's voice. My attempted words of comfort sounded forced and hollow. For me, this was uncharted territory. How – with what words – do you reach someone you love, someone whose heart you know is breaking? All I could say with conviction, the only thing that rang true, was that I loved him, and I always would, whatever happened to either of us.

While I jumped through academic hoops for another forty-eight hours, Dave and his father sat vigil at Pat's bedside. The details he gave me were sketchy. Sometimes, mid-exam, I found myself thinking of this woman I had known so briefly yet come to love so strongly. She had welcomed me, her only child's new girlfriend, with a warmth and sincerity that took my breath away. She was the kind of woman who started buying Christmas presents in January, hiding her cache in the wardrobe until there was barely room for clothes and, by autumn, reindeer-wrapped packages were beginning to tumble on to the carpet. I could see her in Dave's eyes and smile and, most of all, in his values. Basic, simple decency, treating others with kindness, being polite and forgiving, assuming the best in those around us.

Acutely aware of my own limitations – at this stage of medical school I had only learned theory – I reached out instinctively for Dad. 'Just be there for Dave,' he told me. 'You can't make it better, you're not Pat's doctor, but you can make sure he knows he's not alone.'

The moment my last exam was over, I caught a train to Dave and the hospital. At the station, he looked ragged and haunted, with the battle-wearied air of a soldier fresh from action. A man of action himself, of course, but impotent now, unmanned and hating it. Ray, Dave's father, was the same. Between them, they had sat at Pat's bedside day and night, and they were exhausted. I offered to sit with her that night, allowing them some much-needed rest.

When we arrived at the hospital, Dave smiled at his mother. 'Look, Mum, Rach is here.' The faintest of smiles was reflected back at us. Beneath the tubes, cannulas, oxygen and gown, more than anything I was struck by Pat's tininess. Had she always been this small? 'Are you happy for Rach to sit with you tonight?' he asked her.

'Very happy,' she managed to murmur.

I think I knew from the moment I saw her that Pat was dying. Not through any training – biochemistry textbooks are mute on matters of mortality – but through what was *not* there, more than anything. So much life had already taken flight. What was left, the woman lying still as stone on the bed, was using every ounce of her strength not to vanish completely. The act of living was taking everything she had.

Had I known more about hospitals, how wards actually worked, I would have understood that her location in a side room signified her nurses had formed the same opinion. When staff recognise someone is dying, they will do their utmost to find the patient and their family some privacy, if – and it's a big if – bed pressures permit this.

Alone with Pat and my ignorance, I talked to her softly. About our imminent wedding, about Dave's mystery honeymoon plans, about the softness and swish of my dress. Occasionally, I saw the glimpse of a smile. She managed once or twice to squeeze my hand.

'He loves you so, so much,' I told her quietly. 'And you know, I see you in him, every single day. What a wonderful man you and Ray have brought up.'

She opened her eyes and looked directly into mine, as I desperately searched for the right thing to say. How do you comfort? What can possibly make this better? Lost for words, I clung, for a moment, to the warmth and weight of her living hand in mine.

'Pat, I . . . I know you are very ill, but the doctors are doing everything they can. And, whatever happens, Ray, Dave and I are here, we won't leave you.'

She patted my hand, as though it was me, in that moment, who really needed comfort, and I was not sure I had ever encountered a more generous act.

While she slept, I crept out and called my father. 'Dad, Dad, she's dying. What can I do? I don't know what to say.'

'Does she seem frightened?' he asked me.

'Well, no. No. She seems calm.'

'That's very important, Rachel. Make sure she's not in pain, and make sure she isn't frightened. There is morphine and midazolam, if required. They can help. Call me whenever you need to, Rachel, it doesn't matter what time it is.'

That night, I became a human conduit for my father's wisdom. He became Pat's doctor, once removed.

The hours ticked by and things started to change. As her

body began to shut down, I had to step up. In the shadowy hinterland of a hospital at night, where nothing will happen unless others deem it imperative, Pat, without a voice, needed an advocate. First, I noticed her wedding ring was digging into the flesh of her increasingly swollen hand. 'Ask the nurses to cut it away,' Dad advised me, but when I did so, they told me there were no cutters on the ward. Another phone call. 'Look,' said Dad, 'tell them every A&E has cutters for precisely this reason. They can go and get them from there. Or you can offer to go.'

I persisted. Finally, a nursing assistant came to the bedside and, with great skill and tenderness, managed to ease the ring away in one piece, without any recourse to cutters.

Pat became restless, pulling at the oxygen tubes on her nose, fingertips fluttering. The nurses insisted they stay on. Furtively, I called Dad again. 'Take the oxygen off. Unless she's actually bothered by being breathless, just let her rest in the way that makes her most comfortable.' Freed from the plastic, she again slept fitfully.

Now pain seemed to be making her stir.

'She needs morphine,' Dad told me.

'She's on morphine,' I told him.

'What dose?' he asked.

I knew nothing about doses. Hers was the smallest possible, 2.5mg – the same pain relief offered by one small tablet of codeine, and the starting dose of ultimate caution. 'Please,' I begged the nurses, 'get the on-call doctor. She needs more morphine. Please get them here.'

I was, I have no doubt, an infuriating relative. But my fear that Pat might suffer more than was necessary brought out a ferocity I had not realised was there. Eventually, a harried junior doctor arrived on the ward. More morphine was prescribed. And now Pat slept beautifully. I sat and watched the rise and fall of her chest, stroked her hand, smoothed her hair from her brow.

Shortly before dawn, a nurse surprised me with a mug of tea. Far from being accusatory, her eyes were kind. 'If it was my mum, I'd want someone like you looking after her,' she said as she left the room.

As morning activity swept through the ward, Dad had told me precisely what to do. 'Get the palliative care team, Rachel. Make sure they come straight away.' Pat's consultant surgeon hovered briefly in her doorway, itching to be on his way. He muttered vague assent to involving palliative care, backing out of the room even as he spoke. 'No,' I stated flatly. Then, a pause that I hoped was full of steel. I looked him straight in the eye. 'You need to call them now.' I followed him out of the room and stood at the nurses' station, waiting until he picked up the phone. Was I obnoxious, a relative from hell? Perhaps. But if Dad had been her doctor, he would have made the call already, and he was my benchmark, my beacon of good care.

Dave arrived. Safe in the knowledge that the palliative care team were on their way, we swapped places, and I went home to sleep. A few hours later he came into the bedroom. I knew before he spoke that she had died. Tears, the tightest of embraces, no words. For a long time we lay in each other's arms while outside the sky slowly darkened. Four days from diagnosis to death, his mother gone.

Later, Dave described how the palliative care team had carefully, efficiently appraised the situation, treating Pat, now unconscious, with solicitous care. They had started a syringe driver to deliver small doses of drugs, a background infusion to keep her pain-free and calm. In that state, breathing peacefully, with no hint of distress, she had died in her husband's arms.

As for Ray, like his son, he was spent. That day, through his tears and inability to eat, I learned something new about love. That losing a loved one hurts precisely as much as it should do. That the dimensions of Ray's pain, his grief, were exactly what his wife was worth to him. In this mortal arithmetic, she cost him as much as she had mattered, which was to say, boundlessly. I looked across to Dave, who stood at the kettle, pouring tea for his Dad, and I saw with utter clarity that one day he or I would do this to the other, and that I would not for one second wish it differently.

After the funeral, which was swift and shocking – Dave and Ray moving like swimmers mired in treacle, vacant and slow – I took to the fields with my future husband. We set out aimlessly, our strides without purpose, simply putting space and time between ourselves and his loss. The stillness, after the intensity of ritual and condolence, felt eerie, almost other-worldly. It was midsummer, the midst of a heatwave, and the grass in the fields had been solar-torched brown. On and on we walked across mud caked hard as concrete, as the sun slowly stooped towards land. Late now, perhaps eight or nine o'clock, and Dave finally began to talk a little of his mother. We paused on a ridge to look down upon the setting sun. Below us, the field fell away into a sky that was almost uncanny with colour. Pink, purple, green, orange, too luminous, surely, to be entirely natural: a mash-up of dusk with the paranormal.

And then, as we stood, feeling weirdly blessed beneath light far too radiant for farmland, in the furthest limit of my peripheral vision, a ghost appeared. Not a spectre, not Pat's presence, but a ghost owl, a night owl, out on the prowl. 'Dave,' I whispered, and we both held our breath as the barn owl coursed in silence, a head-down hunter, across its dominion of wilted grass. Tilting and swerving from one wing tip to the other, a soporific fighter pilot, trawling languidly for prey. Speechless, we watched as it skimmed the field's breadth, the closest flight can be to a saunter. Approaching the hedge, it turned a wide arc to retrace its flightpath, glowing gold beneath an incandescent sky.

If ever a creature can cross different realms it is the barn owl, a night flier who hunts and haunts by day, who stands still as a gravestone in treetops, who is invariably glimpsed as it fades into darkness, melting back into its gloom. That one should appear in daylight, on this day of all days, dipped in gold under a sky aflame, was enough to make an atheist believe in God or magic.

Then, the owl was gone, the spell broken, and we found we were laughing like children, perhaps in relief, perhaps in something close to awe. How much more remarkable, in the absence of belief, that sheer chance could have given us this daylight ghost, a gift of life from the natural world, of irrepressible life marching on. We embraced beneath the setting sun and then, hand in hand, began the long walk home.

At the time, I chose to bury those ninety-six hours. The shocking nature of sudden loss – here today, gone tomorrow – was too bleak to dwell on and too close to the world of the hospital. All I cared about was trying to support Dave and his father. Yet, as a doctor, unknowingly, my fate was sealed. There was the absolute vulnerability of Pat, her desperate need, during the last night of her life, for a doctor to whom she mattered, someone who cared that those final hours were as comfortable and dignified as possible. And there was the palliative care team, swooping in after dawn, armed not just with expertise but also the conviction that even – perhaps especially – in the last throes of life, superlative care is crucial. This was medicine at its very best, placing patient, not disease, centre stage.

5

Black Wednesday

At a cardiac arrest, the first procedure is to take your own pulse.

Samuel Shem, *The House of God*

'Rach, can you help me?'

Sometimes it is a colleague's tone, more than their words, that signifies the need to drop everything. Caroline, despite being only three months out of medical school, has impressed everyone on the team with her poise and composure. Now, though, she looks wide-eyed and vulnerable, and her voice is taut with anxiety.

I have been a doctor for two or three years now, long enough to recognise that something has gone terribly wrong. As we walk in haste towards her patient, she tries to sketch her dilemma with precision, but the words come tumbling and scattering. 'I think he's about to die. I – I think he might arrest, but at the moment he's for full resus.' She pauses, takes a breath, then blurts: 'And he shouldn't be. He really shouldn't. But when I tried to raise this with the consultant on this morning's round, he just said "no purple form".'

Instinctively, having filled these shoes myself before, I can imagine precisely how knotted and churning she is inside. I'm relieved she has asked for help. DNACPRs – do not attempt cardiopulmonary resuscitation orders – are notorious for their absence inside a patient's notes. Too often, medical teams can shy away from the difficult but vital conversations with patients and their families that help them frame their views on whether they would wish for CPR in the theoretical event of a cardiac or respiratory arrest. The forms are often purple, or sometimes edged in scarlet, because, in extremis, when a patient suffers an arrest, precious moments cannot be squandered scrabbling through some tattered notes to establish the patient's resus status. The form – if it exists – needs to leap out at staff.

In its absence, the default is resuscitation. A crash team descends like a tempest, pumping the chest, shocking the heart, slugging in the adrenalin, doing whatever it takes to try and claw back a life interrupted. Resuscitation is violent, bone-crunching work. During CPR, a dead body is essentially assaulted by a team of doctors who hope to achieve its resurrection. But if that hope is in vain from the outset – perhaps because the patient is too elderly, frail and overwhelmed with illness ever to stand a chance of having their heartbeat restored – then the ending it inflicts is invariably ugly, brutal and devoid of dignity.

Caroline, for all her inexperience, has sensed how precariously her patient is teetering between life and its extinction. For weeks she has cared for him daily, intimately, and today she has discerned a step change in his health. She has accurately diagnosed dying. Despite being batted away by her consultant, she is recoiling at the prospect of her patient enduring the affront of inappropriate resuscitation.

I am only just grasping the rudiments of the case as we rush into Mr Woodman's room. I have never met him before. A man in his late eighties, wizened, skeletal and prone to falls, he has lived for some time with chronic heart failure. In place of strong and synchronised beating, his heart is erratic and bloated, its muscle overstretched and ineffectually pumping. Blood that once pulsed with vigour through his body is now sluggish, with a tendency to pool in his legs and lungs, leaving him waterlogged, swollen, gasping for air. Chronic heart failure has a lamentable prognosis, with between 30 and 40 per cent of patients dying in the first year after diagnosis. During Mr Woodman's stay on the ward the team has tried every combination of drugs to help him, but treatments have essentially run out for him.

His eyes, as they meet mine, are huge and pleading, his face a rictus of pain and fear. I have to fight for a moment to efface my emotions, worried I may reflect straight back towards him the horror that emanates in every direction.

'Help me,' he gasps. 'I'm dying.'

He knows. This is a man enthralled by the certainty that he is now, this moment, on the brink of death. As a student, I was taught early on to beware the symptom of *angor animi* – Latin for the sensation of saturating doom that accompanies the conviction you are dying. At this stage in my career I have encountered *angor animi* only a handful of times, but each has been unmistakable. Mr Woodman's pulse is racing, his blood pressure has crashed, and his lips are stained deep, deoxygenated blue. He has probably just suffered a myocardial infarction – a portion of his heart, abruptly deprived of its blood flow, is dying even as we speak.

There is no time to waste. If death is indeed inevitable, then the kindest – the only – course of action is to obliterate Mr Woodman's terror with sedation, a large dose of morphine or midazolam mainlined into a vein as quickly as possible. But the most senior doctor to see the patient today, the consultant with ultimate responsibility for his care, has prescribed quite the opposite – chest compressions, electric shocks, the full circus of CPR, if necessary. Arguably, even now I should be sprinting to put out a crash call.

Yet from my view, at this moment, from the end of the bed, all of that feels like a travesty. This is a bold call. In the hierarchical world of hospital medicine, overruling your consultant is seen as transgressive, the height of impudence – and, in general, rightly so, since good judgement in medicine is acquired experientially. Seniority, therefore, counts. I am junior. I do not know this patient. Maybe I have missed something glaringly obvious. I think quickly, thoughts careering, trying to weigh all the options.

'Caroline, run and get the boss. Just tell him he has to come now, it's an emergency.'

Next, I ask the nurses to run and draw up ten milligrams of intravenous morphine. Then – the swiftest and least painful way I can think of to prove to the consultant that CPR is wholly inappropriate – I draw a thimbleful of blood that we can analyse instantly. Its biochemistry, I am certain, will prove the utter futility of anything but palliation. But my needle makes Mr Woodman groan and flail. Instead of helping him, as he has begged me to do, I am a doctor inflicting pain. As soon as the blood gas results are back, I have decided, we will give the morphine come what may, and erase the horror, irrespective of whether the consultant is here. It is a plan of sorts, a botched, least-worst compromise. Yet events swiftly overtake us.

As someone runs with the blood to the gas machine for analysis, I am left alone with a dying man. Until the morphine arrives, medicine has nothing, any longer, to offer. All I can give is my humanity. I embrace Mr Woodman, wrapping my arms around his clammy shoulders, and he grips my hand so tightly I almost yelp in pain. He cannot speak now. His face is darkening, clouding. The trickle of blood from where I have punctured his wrist looks impossibly bright on the bed sheets. I try to talk slowly and soothingly, words of comfort and connection, so that he knows, even here on the precipice, that he is not entirely alone. As heartfelt as any I have ever uttered, these words of mine are entirely dishonest. He is going to die, I know it.

A nurse bursts through the door with the syringe full of morphine. Mr Woodman shudders and gasps. His whole body, drenched with sweat, tenses in my arms, face flushing deepest purple. Now the consultant, with Caroline, arrives at the bedside. But his opinion is superfluous, the moment has passed. All of us stand before a man whose eyes are glazing over, and instead of a person, it is a corpse I now cradle in my arms.

For a moment, no one speaks. Silence invades the room like sulphur. The door swings open once more. Another nurse, out of breath, with the print-out from the gas machine. She reads aloud a string of catastrophic numbers, the evidence I had needed to defy my consultant. Too late. The sheets are soaked with a dead man's sweat. We, his doctors, have just failed him.

That night, back at home, many hours between myself and Mr Woodman's death, I still felt bruised by the guilt of failing not one but two individuals. I had put the children to bed, grateful for their distracting vivacity, but now the house was silent. *Angor animi.* My patient had died in terror. Had I been braver, more willing to act on instinct, I might have been able to obliterate his anguish, to becalm the final, fear-stricken moments of his life. But I didn't.

And then there was Caroline, who had run to me for help, hoping to avert precisely this manner of his dying. Afterwards, in a side room, clasping hot tea in her hands, she had wept as we talked about what had just happened. Anger swelled inside me as I looked at this earnest, distraught young doctor, wanting to shout with frustration at the consultant: 'How – *how* – could you have blindly ignored what this patient so obviously needed on your ward round?'

Now, slouched on the sofa, I considered more dispassionately my unvoiced, kneejerk, rhetorical question. Not only had Mr Woodman been given no invitation to discuss his views on resuscitation, the matter of how to proceed in the event of his deterioration had been brusquely dismissed, despite a team member voicing their concerns – the junior doctor who knew the patient better than anyone.

Modern CPR is a brutal, undignified process that was never intended to be performed on patients who are dying from an irreversible condition – such as, in this case, end-stage heart failure. Even among healthy patients, chest compressions and electric shocks – the mainstay of CPR in adults – are often unsuccessful. Only one in five people who arrest while in hospital survive to discharge. For patients who arrest outside hospital, an even smaller proportion – one in ten – survive.

CPR is worth attempting because the prize is survival.

However, the prolonged lack of oxygen during cardiac 'downtime' risks leaving patients alive yet permanently brain-damaged, inhabiting a twilight world in which they have been stripped of their former personality for good. Some people, including me, regard this prospect for themselves as a fate worse than death.

DNACPR discussions allow patients to consider pre-emptively whether or not they wish for CPR. Their wishes, noted in their patient record, help guide clinicians in an emergency, when the patient no longer possesses the capacity to decide for themselves. The purple form is vital in ensuring that, in extremis, it is the patient's wishes and not their doctor's second guesses that take centre stage. So long as they possess the capacity to make the decision, a patient can pre-emptively reject CPR at any time.

Mr Woodman was desperately frail, emaciated and living on borrowed time, having outlived by many months the typical life expectancy for someone with his kind of heart failure. Evidence shows that frailty and comorbidities are associated with worsening outcomes after cardiac arrest, and, therefore, that attempted CPR in these patients has little prospect of success. Why, then, had his hospital team not even broached the subject with him? How, instead, had he been left to die in agonised limbo, a junior doctor floundering at his bedside, compelled by lack of interest by senior staff to act in ways that violated her every instinct for good care?

The answer lies in something murky and strained: doctors' relationship with our patients' deaths. There is a distinct medical unease with, and shying away from, the ubiquitous business of human dying. Society may have outsourced mortality to professionals these days, but that does not mean the professionals necessarily like it.

The failure to conduct vital conversations about CPR is sometimes attributed to lack of time, to too few staff – and overstretched working conditions are undeniably relevant. But deep down, what drives my profession's caginess is, I am certain, a failure of nerve. In spite – or perhaps because of – our medical training, doctors, just like non-doctors, can find talking about death awkward and daunting. Changing this phenomenon for the better requires first an understanding of its causes.

Like anyone reasonably well acquainted with prime-time television, my first impressions of CPR were acquired neither from medical textbooks nor hospital wards, but from the heady excesses of the medical box set. As an avid consumer of *ER*, *House*, *Casualty* and *Grey's Anatomy*, my youthful, pre-medical-school self made the understandable error of assuming that resuscitation tended to be the prelude to steamy romps in an empty on-call room, was delivered by rugged middle-aged men and svelte young women clad in figure-hugging scrubs, and, of course, enabled doctors to showcase their superpowers by heroically saving their patients' lives.

I therefore entered medical school under the blithe and stunningly inaccurate misconception that if I too could be as serene under pressure, as fearless and adroit at pumping a chest, my patients would also pull through. Even after I started traipsing the wards as a fledgling medic, no one taught me how infrequently, in the real world, patients who underwent CPR actually survived to leave hospital, nor how grossly television exaggerates those chances of survival. The so-called 'television effect' – over-optimistic depictions of CPR on screen skewing public perceptions – is well documented in medical research, and affects newly minted doctors as well. I started out presuming that, as per the TV drama scripts, when it came to CPR, everything hinged on me. If I was good enough, the patient would survive. If they didn't make it, the blame was mine.

'It's as simple as A, B, C,' we were once taught, as medical students, by a junior doctor whose eagerness to produce a crack squad of resuscitation protégés had unfortunate repercussions. 'All you need to do is assess the Airway, the Breathing, and then the Circulation,' he stated briskly. 'Just move on to CPR if you can't detect an output.'

'But, what if,' we longed to, though dared not, ask, 'what if the reason we can't find an output is because we're too inept? What if we get it wrong?'

Our instructor had already warned us that if we didn't break several ribs while pumping the chest, we would certainly be failing. Worse still, he told us, with disconcerting relish, 'If you don't do it properly, the patient's brain will be mush even if you do get a rhythm back. Your crappy compressions will have seen to that.'

My first practical foray into resuscitation thus came with the uncompromising message that if I did it right, I would be breaking my patient's bones, and if I did not, I would inflict irreversible brain damage.

I remember us clustering nervously around our CPR mannequins, taking it in turns to save the life of a rubber torso lying, heart up, on a sour-smelling gym floor. Usually, the only heroics here came courtesy of the university badminton team.

The doctor scrutinised our clumsy efforts, scowling from the sidelines and barking real-time feedback.

'No! No! Too slow. Too wimpy. Your elbows are bent. How are you going to transmit any force that way? Why can't I see you sweating?'

Mainly, what I took from this teaching session was an unhealthy dose of performance anxiety. Determined to overcome this, I seized every opportunity to practise. When, as a student, a patient arrested in the bay next to mine, I could not believe my good fortune. At last, I joined an actual crash team for the very first time – an extra pair of hands to swap in and out of the physical labour of delivering chest compressions. The doctor running the arrest appeared effortlessly calm, directing her team with quiet authority and the patient was successfully resuscitated. Transfixed, I watched her every move, wanting to acquire that serenity under fire.

From day one of life as a doctor, cardiac arrests became an integral part of my job. I carried the crash bleep every few days, and all through my nights and weekends on-call. I craved the crash calls, sought them out, hunted them down. I regarded each as an opportunity to become better, more confident, more relaxed at the bedside, learning to direct the high-stakes activity that just might, on those elusive one-in-five occasions, allow the patient to leave hospital alive.

Nowhere in all this single-minded effort to master a technical skill was the patient. Every arrest, I was too busy trying to reinvent myself as the calm, reliable leader of a crash team to really consider the person being battered beneath our interlocked palms. If I am brutally honest, those early crash calls were all about me. My all-consuming urge to get it right, to accomplish it.

And, in one sense, you could argue, that is really not so bad. Should a family member of mine suffer a cardiac arrest while in hospital, I want only one thing at their bedside. Cold, hard, technical prowess. I want a team that launches into action without batting an eyelid. Any hint of panicking or blundering or flapping at the scene and my loved one is less likely to live. I do not want humanity if it comes cloaked in indecision. I want ruthlessly competent doctors and nurses because the longer a heart ceases to beat, the less likely it is ever to start again. So, give me the closest human version of a machine at the bedside. The alternative – the messy, muddled, slow-car-crash dithering I have witnessed, on occasion, as an inexperienced crash team unravels – may just cost my beloved their life.

We make paradoxical demands on our doctors. We want them human, empathetic, caring – but only up to a point. We also want the detachment that enables them to swoop to a crisis – the stopped heart, the mangled limbs, the child suffocating before their eyes – and crack on, undeterred, all instincts to recoil suppressed.

One of the most uplifting moments I have ever witnessed in medicine concerned CPR on a child. Even now, the memory fills me with awe.

As a medical student on attachment in the emergency department, I happened to be in the resus bay when news came through that an ambulance was inbound, bearing an unconscious child.

'What do we know?' asked the consultant paediatrician upon entering the bay, summoned by a paediatric crash call.

'She's called Gemma. She's three years old. She fell into a

canal,' said a senior nurse. 'By the time her parents managed to get her out, apparently she'd already stopped breathing.'

'Paramedics three minutes away,' called another nurse, holding the scarlet phone on which emergencies were always called through to the department.

With a grace and efficiency akin to choreography, a team of professionals who moments beforehand had been as disparate as atoms, dispersed across the hospital, were poised around an empty resuscitation bed, waiting as one to swing into action.

The consultant leading the crash call quietly confirmed each team member's role. The anaesthetist, responsible for airway. The scribe, who would note down, in meticulous detail, the timings, the drugs, the doses, every iota of care which, if we were lucky, might snatch life back from lifelessness. Doctor 1, doctor 2 – the roles and responsibilities went on. Then, a moment of silence before the paramedics' brute force pushed a trolley through the swing doors and there, tiny, limp and pale, lay a toddler, unmoving beneath the harsh fluorescent lights.

It was impossible to hear the paramedics' handover above the screams of Gemma's mother.

'Save her!' she pleaded, over and over. 'Please, please, save her!'

Gently, a nurse discussed with her whether she wished to stay or leave the bay for a moment. The crash team worked on, its focus absolute. In moments, the child had been intubated. Tubes and electrodes sprouted everywhere. Tiny, toddler-sized chest compressions continued, interrupted, like clockwork, every two minutes to check for the resumption of a heartbeat.

Too inexperienced to help, I hovered on the periphery, trying not to wear my shock visibly. I had never before seen a child this unwell. Unless the crash team managed to restart the heart, I was watching, effectively, a dead little girl. I thought of my own toddler, safe at nursery, and of the magnitude of the horror with which Gemma's mother, sequestered in a relatives' room, must now be seized.

On and on the crash team worked. Compressions, adrenalin, electric shocks, compressions. A miniature mannequin, man-handled with conviction. The collective will in the bay for this child to live, to survive, was so strong as to be almost palpable. A forcefield of longing around the bed. Its silent incantation: come on, come on, come on, come on.

Fifteen, twenty minutes must have passed. The resuscitation attempt was going nowhere. In an adult, the risk of brain damage is high, but Gemma's youth gave her body resilience. I bit my lip to keep tears at bay. And then, impossibly, before our disbelieving eyes, the chaotic scrawl of the ECG trace was jolted by the latest shock into something that coalesced into a normal rhythm. Gemma's stunned, battered, fibrillating heart had somehow started to beat again. This body's submersion in brackish water, these lungs fully flooded with rank green canal – despite it all, this little heart had maintained its capacity for life, its inner pacemaker lived. A resurrection had occurred. Right there, on crumpled NHS cotton, a girl had been brought back from the dead. I wanted to cheer to the rooftops.

Not for one second did the team's concentration dip. The luxury of jubilation was forbidden while her life, her brain, still hung in the balance. ROSC – return of spontaneous circulation – is only the first step from an arrest back to health, and Gemma was whisked straight to the paediatric intensive care unit.

The smiles in the resus bay after she departed could not have been any broader. Consultant hugged staff nurse hugged student, in a rare moment of shared elation. But what stayed with me, as I walked out of A&E that night, was not this eruption of joy but its preceding, ruthless dispassion. That total focus while I, on the sidelines, had fought not to quiver and cry. The crash team, simultaneously human and robotic, crunching through the protocols that maximised a child's chances of life. I wanted to eradicate my human weakness and become, like these doctors, part-machine.

CPR, when it works as intended, is nothing short of miraculous. It reclaims patients from the brink of extinction, snatches life from disaster. But three-year-old hearts rarely stop beating. It is the frayed and scarred organs of our elders that more usually, and predictably, give way. At some point, in all of us, cardiac arrest ceases to be a reversible state and becomes instead the natural and inevitable moment of our dying. Our heart stops because it is time for us to go. CPR in these cases is at best pointless, at worst a grotesque indignity.

A fundamental challenge for doctors, therefore, is distinguishing those who can be saved from those in whom the cessation of a heartbeat is the irreversible point of death. Yet at no point in medical school did anyone discuss with us this vital and difficult task. Nor were we taught how to ensure a patient's wishes are at the forefront of decisions concerning CPR. Nor, most fundamentally, *how* to conduct these delicate, all-important conversations with patients and their families. The focus was exclusively on the doing.

In microcosm, the manner in which I was taught CPR

represented the rest of medical school. I was force-fed facts about diseases, not people. Conspicuous by their absence were, ironically, my future patients. I may have filled my brain to bursting with names, numbers, drugs and diagnoses, but I was taught next to nothing about the muddled, uncertain, inconsistent, illogical, forgetful, fearful, frightened, doubtful, real-life flesh-and-blood people who, just like me, inhabited a nuanced world of endlessly shifting grey, not the black-and-white certainties of my medical bookshelves. Overburdened with the insurmountable task of fact acquisition, I found that the entire *raison d'être* of medicine – the patients – was pushed away into the shadows. Which meant, as I approached my first day as a qualified doctor, I had no idea how little I knew.

Every year on the first Wednesday in August around seven thousand brand-new doctors take their first faltering steps on to the wards of NHS hospitals. As if their anxieties are not high enough, a tabloid or two can be guaranteed to recycle lurid claims about the date marking the start of the annual hospital 'killing season' – a spike in death rates allegedly triggered by the fumbling ineptitude of newly qualified young doctors. Whatever you do, some medical wags like to joke, do not get sick on Black Wednesday.

In my case, it felt inconceivable that at 8.59 a.m. on this fateful day I would still be an ordinary member of the public and yet, a minute later, through nothing more momentous than the passage of time, I would have undergone a metamorphosis into doctor, with all the expectation and gravity that entailed. Let loose on to the wards, I would now have the capacity not only to save lives but also to end them. A mistake at work might take the form of a typo or a corpse. I was terrified. For months, my internal mantra was relentless: *Whatever happens, Rach, just do not – do not – accidentally kill someone.* There was no room in my head for anything else. I had to be safe at all costs, and that meant keeping everyone alive, come what may. Nuance did not come into it.

At the end of one of my very first nights on-call, I was summoned by the nurses to assess an unwell patient. I rushed towards the ward, her numbers racing round my head, trying to shake away the treacle of sleep deprivation. Blood pressure, abysmal. Heart rate, skyrocketing. Oxygen saturation, life-threateningly low. A perfect storm of physiological insults. This woman's body was deranged, perhaps irrevocably, and I had only been a doctor for a day or so.

As I arrived, out of breath, at Mrs O'Riordan's bedside, her numbers, in the flesh, screamed emergency. She was, like Mr Woodman, clearly a patient in extremis.

At medical school, we had been assured by the doctors who taught us that you could spot a sick patient from the end of the bed. But I had been the kind of teenager who occasionally made tea by absent-mindedly putting teabags in the kettle. I had always feared that the critically ill might somehow pass me by, the one doctor too incompetent to notice them. Not so. A moment's appraisal of the patient before me triggered the kind of sickening, skin-crawling dread that I would later learn to recognise as 'patient on the cusp of death', and still later to mask, then, finally, to ignore while absorbed in the immediacy of crisis management.

She was tiny and shrivelled, a wisp of a thing. Her skin was grey and wet with sweat, her eyes were wide with terror. She used every muscle she possessed to breathe, the sinews bulging on her neck and chest as she fought and writhed to suck in air. Phrases from my textbooks – 'air hunger', 'work of breathing' – were exposed for the vacuous code they really are. Like 'labour' – a woman's body-splitting toil as she fights for her life to give birth – these are words, you discover, of such insipid pallor they scarcely connect with the real world at all. I saw a shocked, desperate, elderly woman on sheets dark with sweat, pleading through her eyes for someone to save her. On the table beside her was a jar of liquorice allsorts and hand-made cards from the grandchildren. The stethoscope round my neck had never felt heavier.

She might have once helped crack the Enigma code, for all I knew. She might have flown single-handedly across the Atlantic. I did not care. All I assembled, as swiftly as possible, were the medical details that might, if I were lucky, guide her treatment. The idea of refraining from attempting to save her life did not even occur to me.

Ninety-five years old. In for pneumonia. A ropey heart before that. A stroke several years earlier. Oxygen, ECG, large-bore cannula, monitoring, an attempt – unsuccessful – at verbal reassurance. Basics achieved, where to go now? Broader spectrum antibiotics? Fluids? Morphine? I suppose ten or fifteen minutes had passed. Her face looked greyer, her breathing had slowed. Secretions clogged her throat like glue. Her eyes no longer seemed to see me. *No*, I wanted to scream. She was clearly worse. I did not know what to do. I wanted Dad here to guide me. He would have known how to save the day, but my incompetence, I believed, was going to kill her.

It was nine o'clock in the morning, the end of my night

shift and the start of morning handover. Downstairs, in the doctors' mess, everyone would be assembling with team banter and coffee. People would be swearing at the computers for not working, someone cracking a joke about NHS IT being terminal. For a moment, I felt a stab of self-pity.

Five years of medical school, all those exams, yet nothing had prepared me for this. I knew, at least, that I needed help, and called down to the day team. A senior doctor soon arrived on the ward, irate at being dragged from the daily team briefing. 'Please,' I begged. 'I don't know what else I can do.' Thirteen hours on-call hit me all at once. The sunlight was too bright after a night spent scuttling down corridors in darkness.

He surveyed the scene for a moment – my dismay, the trail of blood from my cannula, the woman before him noisily drowning. A flash of impatience. The most cursory of assessments. Then: 'Can't you see she's dying? You do know she's ninety-five, don't you?' With that, he turned tail and left, barking over his shoulder, almost as an afterthought, 'Make sure you call the family.'

In that moment, my childhood notions of doctors as de facto heroes were dispelled for ever. Some of them, it turned out, could be complete bastards. The patient's nurse saw the tears in my eyes and took pity. 'She's not aware of anything now,' she told me. 'Look. She doesn't know what's happening.' Mrs O'Riordan's eyes were glazed and unfocused, her breaths now shallow and sporadic. The suck and slosh of the fluids in her throat had subsided into near-silence. The glitter of panic in her eyes had dimmed into insensibility. 'No one could have saved her, Rachel. She was dying before you even got here.' The nurse now turned to the patient, took her hand. 'It's OK,' she whispered, stroking her palm. 'I'm here. I'm right here with you.'

I had to walk away before I started crying. I knew my patient was taking her final breaths even as I turned my back on her. Worse, that this was the hospital death we have all been led to fear: a brittle and lonely body breaking down behind polyester curtains, among strangers and machines. Rummaging through her notes, I searched for a number for her next-of-kin. My call was answered, and I could hear the shame in my voice: 'Hello . . . is that Mr O'Riordan?'

If we really want to understand why doctors are not always blazing a trail in helping patients and their families confront the fact of human mortality, it helps to imagine ourselves under the skin of brand-new doctors, scattered like pinballs across the wards of their hospitals, ricocheting from one human crisis to another, striving and failing to stop death in its tracks, with all the bone-crushing guilt that entails.

Patients, clearly, come first. But no young doctor should be brutalised by their first efforts at caring, not least because this risks twisting and warping them while still very junior, skewing their attitudes towards death and dying. Take Mrs O'Riordan. A ninety-five-year-old woman who now, I can see, from my position of experience, was dying the moment I first set eyes on her, and who was always going to die, whatever treatment I attempted. Had my father, miraculously, been there by my side, he would have instantly recognised the signs of her impending demise, and worked not to save but to palliate her death throes.

Lacking that insight, never having been taught to consider

it, I found myself locked in what was, without exaggeration, one of the ugliest and loneliest experiences of my life. As I fought to save my patient while she drowned in her own bodily fluids, I knew, with utter certainty, that my ineptness was killing her. That if I had studied harder, learned better, known more, panicked less, this slow-motion horror story would not be unfolding. That, unlike the real, life-saving doctors, my inadequate doctoring was lethal. And when I finally walked out of the hospital that day, I never wanted to go back. I hated the sunshine, the gauzy sky, the children in pushchairs, the chatter at the bus-stop; I hated every single one of the innocent, ignorant men and women around me who knew nothing of the feeling that I had killed my patient. All of it made me want to punch concrete.

Every doctor you have ever met will have almost certainly lived through an experience like this. And most of them will never have talked about it. Debriefing, counselling, emotional support – these standard responses to traumatic events are non-existent in most British hospitals. You kill a patient, as you see it, then you burn up with guilt, then you suffer your shame in silence. No one tells you that you are not to blame. No one even notices you are traumatised. Eventually, provided you have not ended up quitting medicine, you accept that the job of a junior doctor is not remotely what you had thought it would be. Patients in hospital often do not get better. They are old and frail, they die in their droves and medicine rarely can save them. It is not your fault. It is the human condition, our stark cold fate, endlessly skirted at medical school. Hardened, toughened up, you follow suit, still eager to please the older, wiser doctors. Secretly relieved, now you too skirt matters of life and death with your patients, just like your seniors have unintentionally taught you.

One of the most intoxicating aspects of learning medicine was becoming a cryptographer of the human body. Flesh, I discovered, could be read like a book. The way someone walked, their lopsided grin, the rash on their cheeks, the size of their pupils – each sight, sound, texture and mannerism was a clue to potential pathology. For a time, as a student, I could not look anywhere without serious illness leaping out at me. That woman on the bus with the unusually round face and multiple bruises, she definitely had Cushing disease. The tall, skinny lad with unfeasibly long fingers, he had Marfan syndrome, for sure. And those barely perceptible slivers of black on the fingertips – so easily missed unless actively hunted down – suggested a life-threatening infection, deep within the valves of the heart, that was showering microscopic blood clots through the bloodstream like meteors, tiny portents of calamity to come. The first and only time I encountered these 'splinter haemorrhages', I knew we would be diagnosing our patient with infective endocarditis – a heart full of pus, essentially – from the look of one fingertip alone.

But the one diagnosis we were never taught – the condition in which I had found Mrs O'Riordan – was, of course, the state of dying. At no point did anyone explain what dying really looks like, or that our patients would often go on to die despite the team's very best efforts. My cardinal mistake at Mrs O'Riordan's bedside had been the assumption – so naive, so foolish with hindsight – that we could all be resurrected, if only our doctors were good enough.

6

A Numb3rs Game

God does play dice with the universe. All the evidence points to him being an inveterate gambler, who throws the dice on every possible occasion.

Stephen Hawking, 'Does God Play Dice?'

Beneath the faint green glow of the nightlight in the corner, my son clasps his tattered bedtime bear as he sleeps, a scruffy scrap of polyester adored beyond reason since birth. Clutched tight to a toddler's ribcage, the toy gently rises and falls with each breath, as though carried by waves on a shore. Finn sighs when I stroke his cheek with my hand, murmuring something half formed I cannot decipher.

Dave and I have been lucky. Our dream of having children is one we have been able to realise. I linger at Finn's pillow, drinking in the stillness, conscious that a frantic dash to the hospital will be the price of these extra seconds at his bedside. By the time I return in the morning, Dave will have already taken Finn to nursery. This will be it, for nearly twenty-four hours. My fill, my fix. He is too angelic to leave. One last kiss. The smell of his hair. Then, running down the stairs in my hospital scrubs, praying the car will start first time. Outside, in the dark, it is bitterly cold, which in the emergency department spells havoc. I gasp as the frost hits my lungs. Tonight is going to be brutal.

Usually, on the drive to the hospital at this time – just before the pubs close, dispatching their customers our way – I will hear a siren or two from the incoming ambulances. Tonight, though, they are silent, just like the night before. I know exactly where I will find them. I park up and feel the crunch of grit beneath my feet as I jog across ice towards the hospital. Sure enough, there they are, the most dismal queue you will ever see. There must be eight or nine of them this evening, nose to tail, all trapped on the hospital forecourt, each with a crew of paramedics and a patient inside – someone in urgent need of a hospital bed, yet stranded in life-threatening limbo, unable to enter the hospital. The beds are simply not there. The hospital is full to the brim and overflowing. Until someone vacates a space inside, not a single extra person can be admitted. Heart attacks, haemorrhages, sepsis, meningitis – anything might be wrong with these blue-lighted patients for whom, we all worry, time may be running out.

Inside, before I even reach the A&E department I pass its human overspill, pouring out along the corridor. More marooned patients, these ones sprawled on trolleys lining the corridor wall, waiting for a doctor's attention without even the dignity of a curtain around them. I hear whimpering and moaning beneath one bundle of blankets, as a middle-aged woman crouches over the trolley, saying 'It's all right, Mum,

I'm here, Mum' to her hidden, terrified, elderly mother. There are shrieks and abuse from the patient next to her. 'Help me, help me, fucking help me, you fuckers!' He is young and wild-eyed, full of fight and desperation. He may be high, drunk, psychotic or deranged, perhaps, by brain tumour. But I am much more concerned about the man one trolley down – silent, ashen, beads of sweat on his brow, not even connected to oxygen. The police are out in force, weaving in between the harried nurses. 'Trolley two's in SVT,' one nurse yells to another, referring to a runaway heart rate that can trigger a cardiac arrest. 'Can you get a doctor out of Resus now?'

The sobbing, shouting, swearing, gasping, complaining, pleading and groaning are a soundtrack from hell, a cacophony of misery. For a moment, I wish I could drag a government minister by the scruff of their neck from their chauffeur-driven car to this corridor of shame, to see for themselves the reality of a health service pared to the bone under the guise of economic 'efficiency'. Instead, I lower my eyes to the floor, partly embarrassed, partly afraid of incurring the wrath of a relative at breaking point before my shift has even started.

At 11 p.m. sharp, I join the fray. There is the briefest of handovers in the goldfish bowl, a glass-walled hub in the centre of A&E outside which, it is evident, the whole department is bedlam. I cheer inwardly on discovering who tonight's boss is. All the consultants in the department are brilliant, but Nick has a particular air of calm under fire that infects even his most junior colleagues. He makes all of us feel that we are one team and we can do this – an exceptionally gifted leader. I am even happier when he assigns me to Majors. Traditionally, an A&E is divided into three. The walking wounded are assessed and patched up in Minors, Majors is reserved for the more seriously unwell who have been brought in by ambulance, and Resus for those whose life hangs in the balance. This winter, however, a fourth category has emerged: the Corridor – so jammed full of patients on trolleys it needs its own dedicated team of doctors and nurses. Some hospital trusts have even started to recruit doctors to work in 'Corridor Medicine' – the very existence of the job the mark of a service in meltdown.

A friend in another hospital, an old hand in A&E, patrols his own Corridor with gritted teeth and foreboding. One night, he calls me in tears. 'It's beyond inhumane,' he mutters flatly. 'I was literally playing God, choosing who will live or die. And we're the world's fifth richest sodding economy.' His hospital, just like ours, was gridlocked with patients. Every single bed was full, including those in intensive care. That meant his Resus – the part of A&E where patients on the brink of death are rescued, if they are lucky – was crammed with desperately sick adults and children with nowhere to go until someone in ITU either died or became sufficiently stable to be transferred on to a normal ward. Whenever a precious Resus bed became free, my friend was assigned the grimmest of tasks – selecting its lucky recipient. 'I had to walk along the Corridor, deciding who was sickest, who was going to die quickest. I was making death assessments. And the insane thing was, I'd see four or five people I thought should be in Resus. At the very least in Majors. But where were these poor sods? On a trolley by the sluice with no monitoring, no oxygen, no doctors, no dignity. It was barbaric.'

Not for the first time, I am struck by a similarity between hospitals and battlefields. We do not, of course, come under fire, but what we see – the bloodshed, the suffering, the extremes of human experience – is so far removed from 'normal' life that only your comrades-in-arms, your fellow frontline troops, understand it. Unless you have been there yourself, on deployment in an overrun hospital, human lives held so precariously in your overwrought hands, how can you know the price it exacts, the subtle, cumulative taint on a soul?

Tonight, I am far too junior to run Resus or the Corridor, but I know that Majors will be flooded with patients in extremis, which is why, perversely, I am here. With a year or so's doctoring under my belt now, I have morphed into an unabashed medical masochist. I have deliberately chosen these six months of emergency medicine for the immersion in life-and-death dramas. I want to test myself, repeatedly, against shock, seizures, anaphylaxis, strokes, haemorrhages, heart attacks, sepsis, until nothing again can fill me with the dread I felt when Mrs O'Riordan suffocated before my eyes. The cardinal lesson I have taken from her bedside is not that hospital deaths are often unavoidable, but that I must keep on seeking out the acutely unwell – those hovering in the hinterland between life and its extinction – until, no matter what the hospital throws at me, I am sufficiently toughened to be as good as anyone at keeping my patients alive.

A&E is where anything and everything happens. The absurd, the macabre, the bizarre, the heart-breaking. Nowhere speaks more bluntly of how precarious life is, or of how blithely we take it for granted. Amid the stabbed, the shot, the broken-boned, the overdosed, the dog-bitten, the knifed, the burned and the impaled, the department has one message, repeated relentlessly – that life is short and impossibly sweet and forever hangs in the balance. A morning's blue skies may frame an afternoon's carnage. It could have been you, the department tells you daily, who missed your footing while cleaning the gutters and now lies broken-backed, legs limp and lifeless. Or who tripped on the kerb to slide under a lorry. Or who watched their child chase a butterfly straight into oncoming traffic. Or who ate a peanut, undeclared in an innocuous sandwich, and now fights for your life with a tube down your throat and air being pumped into your lungs. Or who managed, inexplicably, one Sunday afternoon, to run yourself over with your new ride-on lawnmower, arriving with your arm inside a Sainsbury's plastic bag, hoping the surgeons might reattach it. (I fished a grocery receipt from the bag in question, sodden with blood and bearing no special offers.)

My first patient of the night is young and defiant. At nineteen, Leila had her fill of hospitals years ago. She has brittle asthma, an extreme form of the breathing disease in which attacks are so sudden and severe that the airways can close off with lethal alacrity. Leila, a politics student, has ended up in paediatric intensive care more often than she cares to remember. She has nearly died many times. Now, with three rings through her nose and her jagged pink hair, she's on a one-woman mission to persuade me to let her leave the department.

'OK,' she begins, before I can get a word in edgeways, 'let me tell you straight off that my sats are 97 per cent and my peak flow is 95 per cent of normal. Seriously. You see what those numbers mean? This isn't an asthma attack. This is not how they go. I'm only here because my consultant gets paranoid.'

I cannot help but smile as we begin to negotiate. 'Attack is the best form of defence, right, Leila?' I counter.

Reluctantly, she grins back at me.

I have to concede, though, that everything she says is spot on. Her blood is beautifully oxygenated, her heart rate entirely normal. When I listen to her chest, there is not a hint of wheeze anywhere. Were I unaware of her history, I could only conclude she is a perfectly healthy young woman. What is odd – the only thing that stands out in her story – is that Leila's specialist consultant in another hospital, the one she saw today as an outpatient, insisted she come here to be checked over in A&E. Something must have niggled him, an eminent professor of respiratory medicine, something I am unable to discern now.

I have no real reason to keep Leila in the department, and the scores of patients on trolleys make it hard to justify asking her to stay for even a few hours' observation. Nonetheless, two things cause me to hesitate: her consultant's unease, earlier in the day, and the fact that it is the middle of the night now. I do not like the idea of any scantily clad teenaged girl setting off alone through the city in sub-zero temperatures, let alone one with brittle asthma.

'Look,' I propose, 'how about this as a compromise? Let me keep you until dawn. I know it's a pain, but at least it's warm here, and I will know you're safe. You can get out of here as soon as it's light, I promise. Deal?'

She eyes me up balefully. Seconds pass. I can hear someone faintly sobbing in Resus. Eventually, through gritted teeth, Leila responds: 'I absolutely hate doctors. You always know what's best for the dumb patient, don't you?'

There is something so vehement about this expression of hatred that I find myself, again, almost wanting to smile. But, in a rush, my heart goes out to her. Beneath the rage and defiance I see a girl who is barely an adult, whose childhood has been a harrowing string of near asphyxiations, whose arteries are stabbed for blood by people like me whenever she enters the hospital, who is cannulated, sedated, intubated and ventilated every time her lungs fail her – and who never, ever, has any power, control over or ability to resist the doctors who take over her body. I had been about to warn darkly of the perils of leaving A&E too soon, but think better of it. Leila, at least, deserves frankness.

Breaking the infection control rules to perch on the side of her bed – there are never spare chairs in A&E, and I loathe looming over my patients – I say, 'Leila, if I'm completely honest, I don't know why I feel like this. But if I let you walk out of here, I will spend the whole night worrying whether you made it home safely. And I can't say why. Something made your professor ask you to come to A&E today. Call it a hunch, a gut instinct – definitely not proper science – but he knows you better than I do and now he's got me worried too. I can't make you stay, and I will respect your decision to leave. You choose.'

Leila hesitates, scowls, and then sags on her sheets, resigned to another night of her life surrendered to the hospital.

'Thank you,' I say. 'I mean it. Thank you.'

She is whisked away to an adjacent area of the shop floor, a kind of holding bay for patients too unstable to be discharged overnight yet insufficiently unwell to earn a proper bed upstairs. For a moment I consider writing up my notes where I am, in Majors, but decide on a whim to follow her round to the holding bay, in case she has second thoughts. This snap judgement, a combination of mistrust and maternal concern, might just be the thing that saves her life.

At first, I write to a standard-issue hospital soundtrack – the bleeping of blocked drips, the electric whirr of automated blood pressure cuffs, the jangle of alarms as a heart beats too swiftly or sluggishly, the snores and the groans of patients in limbo, shuffling and fretting under hospital blankets, destined for a night of fitful wakefulness. It takes a while to notice that Leila is wheezing. The unit is dark – I can barely see her notes to scrawl on – and her softly musical efforts at breathing barely register above the background noise. I keep on writing, eager to finish as quickly as possible and see my next patient. One of the nurses hands me a jelly baby – the crack cocaine of an A&E at night, sustaining entire departments. 'Thanks,' I grin, biting its head off. 'My favourite kind of decapitation.'

Finally, what I am hearing connects with my brain. *Wheeze.* I am bolt upright, hypervigilant. *Wheeze*, becoming louder by the second. Rasping and harsh from the far side of the room. In a patient whose chest I listened to not fifteen minutes earlier, hearing nothing untoward at all. Few sounds are more ominous to the medically trained. In brittle asthma, time is oxygen and every second counts. I am halfway across the room before I realise I am sprinting. 'I need help here, please!' I yell, alerting the nurses as I snatch back Leila's curtain. I can just make her out in the shadows, reaching towards me with outstretched hands.

I flick on the light switch to see her eyes bulging – part panic, part the brute force of dragging air into her failing lungs. But something jars. Her face is blotchy and scarlet, her lips are swelling before my eyes. I frown. It makes no sense. Then, sudden clarity. 'Leila!' I shout, needing her attention. 'Leila! Are you itchy?' She nods, desperate, unable to speak.

Her brain is sensing its own cells being starved of oxygen, and animal panic is taking human form in the sweat on her brow and in her irises, white-rimmed with horror. 'Adrenalin!' I shout. 'Someone get the crash trolley!'

This is not asthma, it is anaphylaxis. Something, perhaps a foodstuff or a chemical Leila has just inhaled, has triggered a catastrophic allergic reaction. Her immune system, supercharged to treat this mystery substance as lethal, has unleashed chemical and biological warfare. Histamine is causing her airways to swell. Fluid is leaking from her veins into her tissues. White blood cells are assembling in their hundreds of thousands. Her blood pressure is crashing, her trachea closing off completely. This is shock and awe, an immunological carpet-bombing, indiscriminate and deadly. Physiologically, there is a grim magnificence, alongside the awfulness, of a human body in high-speed meltdown. I ignore it. We are on autopilot, squeezing bags of fluid into veins, injecting adrenalin into muscles and running Leila, on her trolley, straight round to Resus. By the time we arrive she is blue and unconscious, a whisker away from a respiratory arrest.

Nick, to my relief, is there and takes control. He hooks Leila to fluids and oxygen, and floods her lungs with nebulised adrenalin. In moments, she is strung up like a puppet. She looks small. She looks dead. Her punk hairdo is absurd. She is perfect, too young to be blemished or to die. I have never seen human lips look whiter. The whole world, for a moment, refuses to turn. And then, almost as swiftly as the catastrophe unfolded, we are watching a dead girl coming back to life. The doctor's time traveller, adrenalin, is rewinding calamity. Leila's skin begins to colour, to flush with faintest pink. She stirs, groans a little, looks like she may vomit. I realise my heart is beating so fast I have chest pain.

This girl has just been snatched from the edge of a precipice. She teetered, we grabbed her, we watched her nearly fall. The what-ifs rattle at my skull. What if she had been male, or older, or more sensibly dressed, or less acquiescent, more resistant to her doctor's cajoling? What if I had stayed where I was to write up my notes? What if, in future, the next time she is teetering, we are not there, or we screw up, and she plummets away from us?

I never saw Leila again. The demands of A&E in full winter crisis denied me the luxury of sneaking round to ITU, and by the time my shift was over I was too spent to care. But, as I walked in crumpled scrubs back to my car through the frost, I happened to see Nick doing the same. 'You did well tonight, Rachel,' he told me. 'Anaphylaxis. In someone who was meant to have asthma. Perhaps you saved her life.' I grinned. Perhaps he was right. Finally, I felt at home among the seriously ill. The crackle and heat of A&E were intoxicating.

Invariably, in the emergency department, the humanity with which we treated our patients was inversely proportional to their proximity to death. If your heart stopped beating, we would descend en masse, shattering your ribs in our zeal to bring you back to life. If you had been scooped from the tarmac after a motorway pile-up, we would strip you, manhandle you, drill needles through your bones, all the while ignoring your moans and distress, in our haste to correct your life-threatening trauma. In extremis, I reasoned, every second counts. Time cannot be squandered on building relationships with patients.

And yet I marvelled at the times when a doctor or, more usually, a nurse would endeavour to humanise the medical mayhem. A hand squeezed in Resus. An encouraging smile. A few muttered words to the terrified patient. 'You're doing brilliantly.' 'We've got you.' 'We're going to fix you.'

At first, I relished the sheer numbers of patients who poured through our doors – brief encounters, never sustained beyond the length of your shift that day. Being tempered, toughened into hard doctorly competence, was precisely my aim. But as my confidence grew, so did my unease at the industrial dimensions of this human throughput. Doctor? I was a mechanic to malfunctioning body parts. Bish bash bosh. It was organs we patched, not people.

One day, the whole person proved impossible to ignore. Indeed, she would come to haunt me. I first knew Alice by number, not by name. Amid a frenetic medical 'take' – its mechanical bleeping and human moaning, its location a windowless basement in the bowels of my hospital – her numbers, unattached to a name, leapt out at me.

The take is the lynchpin of most modern British hospitals. Anyone who finds themselves unexpectedly stricken with illness must filter through a take – rapid assessment by a team of on-call hospital doctors – to be admitted under the surgeons or, if an operation is not needed, then under the medics like me.

Considering the take is the route through which every new wave of medical inpatients fills the hospital – three takes a day, each of eight hours' duration, 365 days a year – its organisation is surprisingly archaic. No hi-tech computerised system for ordering and prioritising the patients and their needs. Instead, one hand-scrawled, scrappy piece of paper, Sellotaped to a space on a desk in the cramped nurses' office, listing the name, address and salient medical details of the patients under assessment. Usually, doctors being doctors, everything is completely illegible.

In Alice's case, we didn't even have a name. A general practitioner had sent her our way, alarmed by the information contained within her routine blood test. But her name had somehow been mislaid in the process. All I had before me was digits. An age and a blood count, scribbled in biro. Twenty years old, as-yet-unnamed Alice had a haemoglobin of 45, white cells of 2 and platelets a paltry 30. I stared hard.

Doctors are taught early on to treat the patient, not the numbers – never to lose sight of the real person in front of them. But by now I had been a doctor long enough to know that every rule has its exceptions. And these particular numbers, in a patient so young she has barely crossed the cusp of adulthood, prickled like insects down my spine. The diagnosis they threatened was ominous.

Anonymous, I feared, would turn out to have leukaemia. Her blood counts were dangerously low. The bone marrow, ordinarily a factory that tirelessly churns out blood cells, would be fatally compromised by malignant cells, depressing each of the three normal cell lines – red, white and platelets.

The clamour of the take receded for a moment as, beneath the hospital strip lights, I conjured a young woman about to confront cancer at an age when essay deadlines, boyfriend troubles and occasional rogue haircuts were meant to preoccupy her newly minted adult life. If I had just felt a prickle of fear, what order of emotion would be hers?

Determined she would not slip through the cracks on my watch, I set out to locate her.

'Who's this?' I asked one of the nurses. 'Do we have her name yet?'

'There aren't any stickers yet,' came the reply. 'We don't have an ID. Maybe she still needs to be put on the system.'

Trying to stifle my frustration – patients who present with a new diagnosis of leukaemia can slide all too swiftly into life-threatening extremis – I wove through the early-evening A&E chaos to the office in which a beleaguered yet resolutely unflappable receptionist turned the influx of new patients into typed computer entries, each with an all-important hospital ID.

'Oh, yes,' she told me, cheerfully. 'Alice Byron. Only twenty. Young, isn't she? I'm just printing her stickers now.'

'Thank you,' I said, grabbing the sheaf of identification stickers. Armed, at last, with a name, I set off for the waiting room, hoping the first impression I made would reassure more than it would threaten.

I saw Alice before she saw me. It was hardly a challenge to pick out the student in a waiting room crammed with the frail and elderly who typically comprise an acute medical take. No stick, wheelchair, blankets or spectacles, just a young face in the corner, pale and taut, buried in a book and avoiding all eye contact. Her neighbour, the middle-aged man coiled with anxiety, was, I imagined, Alice's father. A life lived in easy oblivion of hospitals was, in all likelihood, about to be over, and I sensed they may already know this.

'Alice?' I asked gently.

Slowly placing her book in her lap, she raised her eyes to mine. Despite the fear and vulnerability I saw there, I noted reassuring signs of immediate health – her alertness and ability to walk unaided to the cubicle, in spite of her ethereal pallor.

When we reconvened behind cheap bedside curtains, hospital had already made Alice seem smaller. The gown, the wristband, the subtle stealing of identity. But though she hugged her knees to her chest, it was with great eloquence that she told me her story.

Alice had limped through the last few weeks of her second year at university, uncharacteristically low and lifeless. Attributing this to frantic activity in order to deliver end-of-term assignments, she had looked forward to returning to her family home and its creature comforts. Once back home with her parents, however, the crippling fatigue had continued, and with it a new propensity for bruises to bloom unexpectedly in the absence of trauma. Finally, too far for too long from her normal self, she had reluctantly booked the blood test that had delivered her into our care.

It was her father who asked the question doctors dread. I had just alluded to the wide range of potential diagnoses that might underlie her symptoms, studiously avoiding mentioning blood cancer.

'I appreciate common things are common,' he said, 'but what is the worst-case scenario?'

I turned to Alice, sitting stiff and upright on the hospital bed, preoccupied with the line I needed to site in order to replenish her dangerously depleted red blood cells. I endeavoured to allow her to control the conversation by explaining that while some people like to know all the statistics, numbers, possibilities, others preferred not to second-guess the future, electing instead to wait and see how things played out. 'I'm not sure what sort of person you are, Alice. How much would you like to know?'

Inwardly, I suppose I hoped she would choose to skirt the rare but life-threatening diagnoses, but, with what I suspected was characteristic directness, she instructed me to be entirely honest with her.

I paused. If Alice was to trust the innumerable doctors who would soon, I feared, be descending upon her, what she needed from me in this moment was candour.

'Well, there are a great many possible causes,' I began. 'Minor things are common, and more serious things are much rarer. The most serious possibility – what we'd like to rule out – is that all this has been caused by a problem with your bone marrow, meaning it's unable to produce blood cells properly. At its most serious, that could be an illness like leukaemia. But right now, we really don't know.'

I watched closely for her reaction. Medical speculation about worst-case scenarios is invariably as distressing as it is futile. In giving names to hypothetical illnesses, however unlikely, doctors can unleash torrential – and needless – anxiety in patients. But, in this case, neither Alice nor her father seemed remotely surprised. Later, as I wrote up my notes, still troubled by whether I had caused unnecessary anguish, Mr Byron came to find me at the desk. It turned out that he and his wife, like so many anxious parents, had already embarked on their own research, scouring the internet at home for answers. Leukaemia was in the forefront of their minds long before I mentioned it, as was a less well-known haematological condition, myelodysplasia, in which, again, the marrow struggles to produce normal cells.

My heart lurched. I was reminded briefly of the long and lethal roll call of diseases with which my own children had, momentarily, been struck down in my mind – the cricket ball to the head that was surely a life-threatening subdural haemorrhage, the swollen knee that was joint-wrecking septic arthritis, the insect bite that heralded full-blown meningitis – and I longed for this too to be a straightforward case of parental hypochondria.

Of course, it wasn't. Myelodysplasia is exceptionally rare in patients of Alice's age, barely a handful of cases in the UK each year – the equivalent of God throwing several dozen sixes in merciless succession, one after the other. Yet, somehow, the Byrons had correctly identified their daughter's diagnosis even before she arrived in hospital.

My shift ended as Alice was admitted from A&E on to a medical ward, and from there to the specialist haematology centre. Though our paths had crossed only briefly and by chance, and I was never to meet Alice again, in my mind her presence lingered. The quiet composure despite the palpable fear, the well-thumbed copy of Harry Potter by her side. Above all, her youth, and the unfairness of it all. A family plunged without reason or warning into hospital hands, whose plight could have been any one of ours.

I had thought that was the end of the matter. Alice, the young woman I knew first as a constellation of numbers, was, if not forgotten, then subsumed beneath the relentless surges of patients that comprise day-to-day acute medicine. Then, several months later, a haematologist friend happened to ask if I was following the young patient's blog everyone was talking about. 'You'd love it,' he told me. 'She's an English student and she's even called Byron.'

'You mean Alice?' I asked. 'I was the first doctor she ever met in A&E. She was so young.'

'Well, you'd better read it then. You're probably in it.'

That night, with the children asleep and the house temporarily restored to a semblance of order, I poured some wine and opened my laptop. There, vividly, was Alice:

I'm nineteen at the beginning of this twisted fairy tale, in my second year studying English Literature at Cardiff University, and I'm pretty damn normal. I have a couple of great circles of friends, several that I'm lucky enough to have known since I played kiss chase and wore my hair in bunches, a wonderful family, a busy but fun part-time job at home, and a quiet appreciation for comfy pyjamas and pretty, pastel-coloured things.

In unflinching prose, with neither pity nor mawkishness, Alice charted her symptoms, her diagnosis, her fertility treatment and the harvesting of her eggs before, finally, inevitably, her myelodysplasia transformed – as she had been warned it would – into an acute leukaemia requiring aggressive, life-threatening chemotherapy. When that moment came, six months or so after she first presented to hospital, she described it with brutal frankness:

After a sleepless night and some fast-tracked biopsy results, my consultant confirmed it today. When I was first diagnosed in June, my bone marrow was made up of only 1% of blast (cancerous) cells. Today, it is made up of 50% of them. My body has been totally, completely invaded, and I'm still trying to wrap my head around the fact that on Tuesday evening I was contemplating where I could book an eyebrow wax, and by Friday I'd learnt that I wouldn't need an eyebrow wax anytime for the foreseeable future, because I was suddenly listening to a doctor spell out chemotherapy regimes and hair loss.

But there it is. In two weeks I won't have any hair. Or functioning bone marrow, for that matter, as the chemo wipes it out bit by bit . . .

I don't know how to feel about having to maybe write some kind of will that leaves my dad in charge of paying off the Amazon debt I've racked up buying Kindle books (I know, I'm wild, somebody stop me), because I still sleep with a stuffed Eeyore and five months ago I was at university, getting my kicks out of wearing a toga to a women's rugby social. This is all new territory for me.

Doctors specialise in kicking their patients in their metaphorical guts – 'the treatment hasn't worked', 'the cancer has returned', 'there is nothing more we can do' – but this time, the tables were turned. Momentarily floored, the mother in me aching, I stopped reading, closed the laptop and poured more wine before resuming Alice's story.

In the end, the young woman I had first encountered as nothing but a clutch of numbers, then slowly come to know and love through the vibrancy of her written voice, was herself drawn to the sheer outlandishness of her own statistics. Alice was the youngest ever patient with myelodysplasia on her ward, the one with the highest ever documented fever, the most virulent cancer, the longest odds. In hospital, it seemed, she broke every record effortlessly, when the last thing you want, as a patient, is to be remotely fascinating in your doctors' eyes. Her final blog, written the day before she received a bone marrow transplant from an anonymous donor – a last-ditch attempt to arrest her rampaging leukaemia – was even entitled 'A numb3rs game':

Today I Googled how many days the average British woman lives for. Morbid, I know, but bear with me on this. She lives for 82.7 years. That's 30,185.5 days. It sounds like a lot, and it is, if you try and forget about all the time we spend sitting in traffic, queuing in Tesco, perhaps cleaning up our children's sick, and how many days menial tasks like that take up.

I did a little calculation of my own, and so far I've been kicking around for 7,682 days. The last year-and-a-bit of those days, however, the last 369, to be precise, ever since that awful day just over a year ago when I got admitted to hospital on the back of a blood test for anaemia, and left, eventually, with a blood cancer diagnosis, have been occupied with words and thoughts such as 'haematological disorder', 'bone marrow transplant', and then 'cancer', too. That's a lot of days wasted to this shitty disease already, and I know that there are many more to come, but tomorrow marks a chance to say goodbye to some of those thoughts. To say goodbye, little bit by little bit, to the worried phone calls from relatives, the hospital stays and the needles and the poisonous drips . . .

It's not over yet, not by a long shot, but all I know is that

I'm tired, most of all, of my days being measured in numbers, in statistics, including a 75% chance of none of this being worth it. But I'm ready to crack on with it anyway. Despite my odds, I want those 61.9 extra years that the average British woman has promised me. I want my life back now, please.

Alice died less than a month after her transplant, shortly after turning twenty-one. There was no respite from the needles and poisons. In striving for the sixty-two years of life out of which she had been cheated, Alice endured another gruelling three weeks of medical interventions until her new marrow, despite everything, failed.

Among non-haematologists, the speciality has a reputation for being guilty of over-treatment. There is a suspicion, perhaps justified, that haematologists strive relentlessly for cure at all costs, subjecting their patients to distressing treatments even though they are doomed to fail. Medics are notorious for our black humour, and the in-joke about haematology goes: 'Why are people buried six feet under?' The answer: 'To make sure the haematologists can't get to them any more.'

Arguably, some of the accusations levelled at haematologists are based upon a misunderstanding of the course of haematological malignancies. Unlike solid tumours, in which cure usually hinges on a surgeon cutting a cancer away before it has had a chance to spread, in blood cancers, the malignant cells are disseminated from the outset, freely coursing through the blood or lymphatic systems. Leukaemias, for example, are often unruly, uncontained, rampant diseases against which the surgeon's knife is futile. The mainstay of their treatment is, instead, intravenous chemotherapy – infusions as elusive and all-pervasive as the cancer, able to penetrate the body's every nook and cranny. As such, the natural history of blood cancers is less predictable than that of solid tumours. With leukaemia, 'Did we catch it before it spread?' is a redundant question. Only with hindsight, when the chemotherapy is unsuccessful, does it become clear its infusion was futile.

More fundamentally, from the patient's perspective, despite knowing very well how bleak her odds were – the meagre one-in-four chance that her bone marrow transplant would save her – Alice wanted every last-ditch attempt at cure. The sheer, demanding starkness of those final words: *I want my life back now, please.* Unless you have been there yourself, is it possible to imagine being forced to confront at the age of twenty – barely a step beyond childhood – the prospect of being cheated out of your entire adulthood? Could a doctor, could anyone, have refused her?

When a patient is as young as Alice, and as desperate to live, pulling out all the stops feels entirely uncontentious. This is exactly when we want our doctors to play God, to hurl everything they have at an illness – to try their utmost to reverse the random throws of the dice, to intervene, to turn the tide, to reclaim life from its premature extinction.

As we age, our vitality wanes but not, necessarily, the ferocity of our desire to live. Treatments may be every bit as keenly wished for, even as our bodies accumulate illnesses and frailties that, together, shrink to next to nothing the likelihood of cure. Andy Taylor, a former BBC television journalist, was diagnosed with another type of blood cancer, multiple myeloma, at age forty-six. Although free from serious comorbidities, Andy's age alone meant that the only treatment capable of eradicating his myeloma – a bone marrow transplant like Alice's – was, statistically speaking, highly likely to kill him. The kinder, gentler, safer treatment options his haematologists encouraged him to consider would buy him more time – up to seven years, if he were lucky – but they could not bestow the cure for which he yearned. He dismissed them without a moment's hesitation. For Andy, it was all or nothing.

'What use were they to me?' he told me. 'What was the point in any of that? I didn't want just a few more years. I had children. I wanted to live. I wanted to see them grow up, go to university, get married, have kids of their own. I didn't want to miss any of it. I wanted it all. Seven extra years were absolutely no use to me. People would say to me, "Gosh, what a difficult decision to make," but I've never found any decision easier. I wanted life.'

Andy's single-mindedness paid off. He surprised his doctors by surviving his gruelling transplant, thus becoming one of the statistical outliers whose very existence inspires hope and, arguably, unrealistic expectations in others. Today, some ten years after his transplant, he is healthy, outspoken and 'every bit as bloody-minded'. He is also living proof that doctors' best guesses about prognosis are fallible, and that patients can defy the bleakest of odds.

Medicine, in short, as Alice Byron described so eloquently, is a numbers game – but one in which the self-appointed games-masters, the doctors, cannot always add up. Like everything else in medicine, predicting life expectancy is fraught with uncertainty, an imprecise attempt to balance risks and probabilities on the basis of incomplete information. There are no crystal balls inside a hospital. In the messy, imprecise space in which doctors can never say never – unable to rule in, or out, a patient's survival with certainty – human hope can soar, take flight. Alice and Andy chose to fight for life at all costs, in spite of knowing how dire their odds were. Intervention, for them, was everything. They wanted to keep going until the bitter end, even if it killed them.

I think – though none of us really knows for certain – that I too, if faced with a life-threatening illness, might wager everything on the high-stakes treatment that would kill or cure. I might badger, harangue and plead with my doctors to have the least reliable, most experimental interventions, if I thought they could protect my children from the pain of losing their mum. The careful, evidence-based, dispassionate reason that guides – or so I hope – my medical decision-making might amount to so much hot air if the only outcome that meant anything to me was the one that made winning the lottery look commonplace.

7

Storytelling

*After nourishment, shelter and companionship, stories are the
thing we need most in the world.*

Philip Pullman

The man widely regarded as the father of modern medicine,
the late-nineteenth-century professor William Osler, famously
recognised the unique importance of stories in medicine. Osler
insisted that medical students and young doctors in training
should learn from seeing and, crucially, from talking to their
patients. Memorably, he said: 'Just listen to your patient, he is
telling you the diagnosis.'

Those words are as true today as they were back then. For
all the high-tech wizardry of modern medicine – the scans, the
genomics, the molecular analyses – it is still the case that invariably, simply by paying close attention to what a patient is telling
us, a doctor can work out their diagnosis. Storytelling – a
patient describing to their doctor their own illness narrative –
is, then, the bedrock of good medical practice.

The author Philip Pullman goes one step further. In boldly insisting upon stories as imperative for human survival – one of the things we need most in the world – he imbues them with transformative force in medicine. It is undeniable that the meanings we construct around our afflictions and diseases, the stories we tell ourselves about what is wrong, and where we are heading, can overturn our experience of illness. But, in the cut and thrust of a busy teaching hospital – the cardiac arrests, the major haemorrhages, the crash calls, the life-and-death decisions being made every hour – you might imagine that storytelling is the last thing on a doctor's mind. We are all far too busy doing our jobs, often with time running out.

Alice Byron's story – her voice clear and true – taught me that Pullman's words are nowhere more apt than in a hospital, where what heals is not confined to a doctor's drugs or scalpel blades. It is the quieter, smaller things too – being held, heard and shown you matter – that make patients feel cherished, and hospitals humane. I see Alice as clearly today as my father remembered the two naval ratings with whom, some five decades past, he talked and joked, and to whom he gave comfort and love as they succumbed to their full-thickness burns. Had any fiction ever mattered more, I wondered, than the one he had tried to give them?

A colleague from one of Britain's foremost cancer hospitals, the Royal Marsden in London, demonstrates the power of storytelling beautifully. A children's play specialist, she set out to tackle the fears and anxieties of children facing radiotherapy for cancer. When the treatment is given, no one else can be in the room, so the child, of necessity, is separated from their parents to face a loud and intimidating machine alone. Sometimes, only a general anaesthetic – a risky procedure, avoided if possible – can quell a child's terror at being abandoned in the radiotherapy suite.

After careful consideration of this matter from her young patients' perspective, the play specialist invented something she called 'magic string': a simple ball of multicoloured twine, one end of which the child could clasp, while the other would weave out of the room, under the door, to be held by their parent. She had devised a literal thread that was, simultaneously, a narrative thread, a story that a frightened child could tell themselves, while lying cold, alone, behind a lead-lined door, that Mummy or Daddy were still there, on the other side, caring and holding on to them. Simultaneously cheap as chips and priceless, magic string helps children with cancer today reframe their experience away from abandonment to being nurtured, loved and supported.

As with any addiction, I found that the hits of emergency medicine, though intoxicating, were unsustained. Life-saving of an altogether more prosaic kind – the myriad ways we can help someone feel human in hospital by treating their story with the respect and attentiveness it deserves – seeped indelibly under my skin. In matters of life and death, I was learning, sometimes actions spoke softer than words.

'Can you come straight away? The Brugada in 3A can't breathe.'

'What's the patient's name?' I asked through a fog of fatigue.

'Name? I . . . don't know. Resp rate is forty, he's on fifteen litres. Due an ICD tomorrow.'

I struggled to hide the irritation in my voice. 'OK. I'm on my way.'

It was 4 a.m., the zombie hour. Seven hours into a frenetic night shift, I wilted at the thought of the remaining five or six. It had been crisis after crisis after crisis. As I hurried the length of the hospital, trying to shake myself free of grogginess, there rose from the darkness a sound of insurgency. Clamouring, chorusing specks of life, sparrows or blackbirds most likely, invisible heralds of the day to come. But their jauntiness, this pre-dawn cataract of jubilation, stirred in me self-pitying rage. *What time do you call this?* I wanted to snarl. *Enough with the euphoria. Can't you keep your joy to yourselves?*

The Brugada in 3A was a man on the cardiology ward, aged forty-one, gasping and writhing in his bed for air. His name was Tom. He supported Manchester City. He loved taking his twin toddlers to the park for a kickabout. But a few months ago, while chasing after his three-year-olds, he had found himself felled, lying poleaxed on grass, staring quizzically up at blue sky.

'Are you all right, mate?' came another man's voice from afar.

Tom had blinked, his forehead creasing into a frown, unable to formulate words. Then he had stirred, gasped a little, struggled to rise.

'Take it easy, mate. You just keeled over. Don't worry. Your lads are right here.'

The twins hovered uncertainly at their father's side. 'Daddy? Daddy?' Four outstretched arms. 'Here, Daddy. You can have the ball now.'

The cause of Tom's collapse, unbeknown to him, was a rare inherited heart condition that predisposed him to fatal cardiac arrhythmias. Brugada syndrome, invisible and deadly, is one of various diseases that can cause sudden cardiac death. One moment, the heart's four chambers are a synchronised pumping machine, the next, and they quiver and flail uselessly as the heart is subjected to an electrical storm, the blood pressure crashing to nothing. Had Tom's heart not spontaneously regained its normal rhythm, he would have been dead in moments.

As it was, he chose to dismiss his unnerving collision with turf as a 'blackout', nothing more than a benign curiosity, certainly not worth worrying his wife about. That night, when she noticed the graze on his arm, skinned on impact and still faintly grass-stained, he made a self-deprecating joke about the dangers of Premiership football. How much easier to reframe the sinister as slapstick.

The next time it happened was different, impossible to ignore. Several weeks later, besuited, caffeinated, wired and jangling from the daily ordeal of the rush-hour commute, Tom arrived at work. He jogged up the stairs, as he had done ever since reading some piece in the paper extolling the benefits of embedding ad hoc interval training into your urban working day. But this time, instead of striding out of the stairwell into his open-plan office, Tom turned himself into the day's hottest gossip, a drama, a spectacle, a public display of infirmity. Even now, even knowing what had caused his second collapse, he could not help wincing at the thought of lying motionless on linoleum in front of his colleagues, of the paramedics pressing him back down on to the stretcher as he sought to rise, of all that eager, insatiable gawping at his diminished state, the golden boy turned lame duck, fainting – *fainting* – and being whisked off to hospital.

The hedge fund in which Tom worked was nothing if not a pure meritocracy. Only one thing really mattered and Tom's knack for profit had dazzled the bosses. He could outperform the algorithms, generate money from air. He was well aware that some of his contemporaries would like nothing better than to see him fall from grace.

I knew none of this when I first set eyes on him. I saw a man in blind panic, clutching his chest and yelling angrily, 'I can't breathe! I can't breathe! Where the hell is the doctor?'

'I *am* the doctor,' I responded tartly, noting Tom's normal blood pressure, oxygen saturations and the vigour of his outburst.

'He was having panic attacks all through the day as well,' murmured one of the cardiology nurses wearily.

My interaction with Tom was brisk and perfunctory. Talking authoritatively, instructing him to mimic his doctor's breathing, swiftly brought his panic under control. The moment I felt satisfied he was safe, I was gone. I did not care what lay beneath his nocturnal terror. I scarcely had time for the real emergencies, as I saw them – the strokes, the arrests, the bleeds, the sepsis – let alone those generated by minds run amok. My callousness, my judgements, were in part the product of bone-crunching fatigue, but also, I knew, a kind of prejudice. When you are stretched too thinly, meanness becomes a survival mode. I had no time at night to indulge neuroticism.

A day or so later, my night shifts over, I met Tom once again on the ward. The cardiologists had fitted an ICD – an implantable cardioverter-defibrillator – beneath the skin of his chest, his inbuilt insurance against sudden cardiac death. Should the electrical pulse in his heart fail again, the ICD would shock it back into life. His very own crash team, a mere three inches wide.

Tom was due to be discharged home the following day and I

needed to ensure he knew when to come back to clinic. It was early evening. I was eager to leave. But this time, I found myself lingering at his bedside. Perhaps I wanted to make amends. I knew my manner before had been horribly peremptory and, as I looked at him now, pale and anxious, I found myself guiltily lowering my eyes.

'Do you mind me asking, Tom, have you had any more panic attacks?'

He stared at me hard, hunting, I believed, for signs of doctorly sneering. 'A couple,' he muttered tersely. 'None as bad as the other night.'

I tried to imagine how it must have felt to be told, while stripped of your identity in a hospital gown, small and exposed beneath strip lights, that your heart, at any moment, could stop beating for ever. That your body, once so healthy it had been merely an afterthought, was now a treacherous, decrepit disappointment. I took a deep breath.

'I'm really sorry I was so curt the other night,' I said. 'I was exhausted. I didn't mean to be dismissive and I shouldn't have been. It was out of line.'

Tom's expression softened. 'Well ... at least you have the decency to apologise.'

I smiled nervously back at him. 'Do you feel any safer now, with the ICD in?'

'Honestly? Not even bloody remotely.' He paused, staring helplessly at his upturned hands. 'I nearly died, just like that. And ... sure, I have this metal box inside my chest now, but so what? I could die from something totally different tomorrow. We all could. And ... what is the point of anything, when you know that?'

'So . . .' I hesitated, trying my hardest to understand him. 'Am I right in thinking that the panic is *not* because you think you're suddenly going to drop dead?'

'Exactly. It's not the dying, it's what the dying means for the living. I mean, it's all pointless. It's all for nothing. In a hundred years no one will even know you existed at all.' He clicked his fingers at me. 'Did you know two people die every second?' Clicked them again. 'There go another two.' Click. 'And another. Me. You. My wife. My kids. Gone. A flash in the pan. Ancient history.'

Tom's panics, it seemed, had been triggered not by the prospect of sudden death, but by his painful new awareness of our inescapable transience – the sheer brevity of human life, a spark, burning briefly, against the maw of deep time – and his craving for something that persisted.

'I feel paralysed by it,' he said, almost guiltily, 'the thought that everything that lives ends up as nothing. What's the point in living at all?'

'Let me ask you a question,' I said cautiously. 'Imagine your boys in a few years' time. Maybe ten or eleven. Old enough to indulge their Dad's existential angst.' Tom smiled and, emboldened, I continued. 'Suppose they said to you, Dad, how should we live our lives when we know we're going to die? What would you say to them?'

Tom weighed this up carefully. 'Well, I suppose I'd tell them about how beautiful the world is, about getting outside and enjoying it, about how much pleasure there is being around people you love, and how, at the end of the day, the small stuff – playing football with your kids in the park on Sunday – is what matters. That kind of thing. You know.'

'Well, there you are then. That's your answer. None of what you've described is valuable because it's permanent. No one says, "What's the point in that sunset? It's just going to be over in a second."'

Tom sat for a moment saying nothing. Eventually, ruefully, he laughed. 'Yeah, yeah, I get it. Basically, I should quit the City and become a hippie, right?'

'Maybe,' I grinned back at him. 'Depends how much you like Porsches, I suppose. But, seriously. All that stuff you love about life, it's the day-to-day flow of it, isn't it? Those moments, as they're lived. Why should something have to last for it to have beauty or value? For what it's worth, I'm such a hippie I think I love things even more *because* they don't last for ever. Maybe we all do.'

Tom walked out of the ward the next morning, alive and protected by the box in his chest, primed to deliver the shocks that would preserve him, for a time, from the human fate of oblivion. I had no idea if our conversation had helped him, but while we had sat side by side as dusk fell, I believed my attempt to understand his fears had conveyed, at least, that his doctor cared about him.

As we had talked, I had been struck by a thought which then had seemed too wildly inappropriate to voice, but which, to this day, I suspect Tom would have found compelling. Suppose he *had* died from sudden cardiac death – instant obliteration, his life erased at a stroke. Ironically, far from confirming life's pointlessness, Tom's very transience would have instilled his life with meaning. For at his post-mortem, most likely, his Brugada syndrome would have been discovered. His own sons could have undergone genetic testing. And so, in dying young, being felled in his prime, he might have saved his children's lives. As legacies go, it is hard to imagine anything more potent or enduring.

Only a few years into my medicine, I saw how fiercely staff were fighting to preserve their instinct for kindness. All around, compassion fatigue was rife. I saw doctors and nurses who had barricaded themselves away from the human beings they tended, becoming hardened and withdrawn, simply to survive.

Nowhere was this more starkly the case than when patients confronted the final experience of their lives. I had thought deaths on trolleys in corridors could not be surpassed for sheer brutality. Then, one day, with tears in her eyes, a junior colleague described her own recent experience of winter. Carly's A&E, as usual, had been stretched to breaking point. Patients were stacked up on trolleys in corridors, bed managers frantically pressuring the medics to turf out anyone capable of staggering home. Carly, still in her first year as a doctor, had never known anything like it.

'I know I don't know about war, but it was what I'd imagine a war zone to be,' she told me. 'I hadn't eaten or had a drink all day. It was chaos.'

In the early evening, a senior manager instructed Carly to escort an elderly patient from A&E to a ward. Obediently, she did as she was told, too exhausted to question why a medical escort was necessary for the frail ninety-two-year-old, alone in a bay, without even a pillow for comfort. Only once the lift doors closed, and she found herself travelling up eight floors with a porter and the patient on a trolley, did she see the wild panic in his eyes. 'He kind of gasped,' she told me. 'His face started going dark and I could see he was dying right there in front of me.'

By the time the lift doors reopened, the patient's heart had already stopped beating. Carly had entered the lift with a person, only to emerge with a corpse. Someone whose dying moments were spent with neither loved ones nor dignity, but instead involved him being treated like a package in transit, more FedEx parcel than human being.

Grotesque as this was, I could see precisely how it had happened. Surrounded daily by the moans and cries of patients trapped on trolleys, is it any wonder staff become sufficiently hardened to shunt dying pensioners into lifts to clear beds for the sick still waiting outside? How else could they keep going on?

I wanted the opposite. I wanted to retain my kindness, my impulse to care, not have it bludgeoned out of me. The spoken word, I had come to realise, could be as delicate and important as any physical intervention, and sometimes equally life-changing. Words are a means through which doctors build trust, assuage fears, signal compassion, resolve confusion, instil hope – and, on occasion, remove it. But they cannot be rushed. Above all, when your focus is people, not body parts, taking time to listen to your patients' words – seeking truly to understand what matters to *them* – can have astonishing potency.

I found myself gravitating towards the difficult conversations that some of my colleagues would go to any lengths to avoid. Revealing a diagnosis of cancer or, worse, that the cancer has returned. Persuading a patient, gently but firmly, to desist from clutching at straws. Looking on as the enormity of loss crumples your patient's face, and they begin to confront death's imminence.

Sometimes, talking felt too close to home. 'I have this patient who reminds me so much of Gramps,' I told Dad one day.

Arthur had spent a torrid time on our ward, after being rushed to A&E scarcely able to breathe. A tall, brawny man in his eighties, he had spent all his life on his farm. The source of his breathlessness was seven decades of smoking. Not, on this occasion, a lung cancer, but COPD – chronic obstructive pulmonary disease – the scarred and tattered, tar-clogged lungs that are the fate of every long-term smoker. Arthur's disease had finally caught up with him. He was prone to back-to-back pneumonias no amount of antibiotics ever quite managed to shift. He ran fevers, lost weight and permanently coughed up thick sputum. For over a year now he had relied on oxygen therapy at home. Rarely, if ever, did he dare remove it.

What reminded me so powerfully of my late grandfather was Arthur's attitude to his family. His devotion to his wife, Beryl, touched us all on the ward, as did his affection for his unruly clan of children and grandchildren. When his breathing allowed it, Arthur loved to describe its youngest members' antics.

'Gemma's been baking for the school cake sale,' he proudly announced one day. 'She's giving the money to the hospital charity. And Tommy's offered to sell his model aeroplanes. They know their granddad is being well looked after here. They say they're going to help other patients too.'

Invariably, as I left the ward in the evening, one or more small children would be clambering over their granddad, oblivious to the oxygen tubing, monitors and sputum pots that encroached on his bed space. His lungs like bellows, sweat on his brow, Arthur, nonetheless, would be beaming.

Initially, he had done well on the ward. Potent intravenous

antibiotics had transformed his breathing over twenty-four hours. We hoped he was set for home. But after that initial rally, he began to decline. Occasionally I would glimpse him from the end of the ward, sitting bolt upright on the edge of his bed, leaning forward with lips pursed and blueish, the muscles in his neck bulging like cords. One day, we broached the matter of morphine.

'People know about morphine for pain, Arthur, but it can really help with the feeling of breathlessness too. A small dose might make you feel more comfortable,' I suggested.

'Morphine?' Arthur repeated slowly. A pause, while this sunk in. 'So . . . you think it's time for morphine, do you?'

I knew – or at least I thought I did – what Arthur was afraid of: that, in proposing morphine, I was communicating a darker truth, that his death was drawing near. And, in truth, I could not have denied this. When someone's lungs are failing so badly that even lying still on a bed leaves you clamouring for air, morphine brings relief to the final stages of lung disease only by suppressing the hunger for oxygen. Its use is a last resort. Nevertheless, with great reluctance, Arthur agreed to testing out a dose or two. To his surprise, he found morphine dramatically helpful. 'Most of all,' he told me, 'it makes it a bit easier for me to chat to the grandchildren. That's what makes my day.'

One morning, I found him looking flushed and sweaty. Beryl, at his bedside, was wringing her hands. There was a gauntness to his cheekbones I had not seen before, new hollows and caverns beneath his eyes. These were the contours of death's approach, flesh one step ahead of its executioner.

I sat down. 'How are you feeling, Arthur?'

'Tired,' he gasped. 'So tired.' A pause. Beryl, head bowed, began to cry. 'It's another infection, isn't it?'

'I think so,' I agreed. 'Your temperature's very high.'

For a while, we simply sat together, weighing how to proceed.

'Arthur,' I began, watching him closely, 'may we please talk about what you would like to happen next?'

Husband and wife exchanged glances.

'We could give you more antibiotics. But ... is that what you would like?'

'We've discussed it already,' said Arthur quietly. 'No more antibiotics. We both agree. No more.'

We talked for a while about how things might develop. How the infection, if virulent, might claim his life in a matter of days. That evening, as I left the ward, I noticed Arthur was alone, chest like a piston, rising and falling, eyes half closed. I hesitated. To my surprise, when he looked at me, I saw the glint of tears. My mind leapt to instant conclusions. *He's terrified. He's grieving. He can't bear to let go.* But Arthur looked my way and smiled. He patted the bed.

'Don't look so worried. Come and sit next to me.'

I moved closer. I could see droplets of sweat on his brow.

'I'm not crying for the reasons you imagine,' he began. 'There is something you don't know. Something no one knows.'

In fits and starts, as his broken lungs permitted, a story emerged of love and forbearance. I found myself holding my breath, even as Arthur struggled to draw his.

'All my life, Rachel, I've been lying. All my adult life,' he whispered. 'But what you have to understand is that I grew up in the fifties. When I was a boy, what I was, it was a crime. Either I lied to myself, or I accepted I was ... a deviant. That was no choice at all.'

I did not move a muscle. I knew I was being handed something precious, profound. A secret so sacred I felt less doctor than priest. Here was a man, reaching out across his death-bed, towards someone he trusted would neither shun nor condemn him.

'I suspected I was a homosexual while I was still at school,' said Arthur. 'I tried to convince myself I wasn't.' He paused. Talking was a losing battle against failing lungs. 'Beryl has been more than any man could wish for. Her love, her heart. But . . . I loved someone else. And I could never tell my family.'

For decades, Arthur had been in a gay relationship. Covert, shameful, a lifetime spent in hiding. I had the sense that he was grieving for the man he had never been able to be, his true self, his real self, stifled by society's prejudices and his personal sense of duty.

'I couldn't be there when he – Jonathan – died. His children were with him at the end, not me. And even if he was still alive today, he wouldn't be able to be with me now. I'm alone.'

Instinctively, I found myself taking my patient's hand. I thought of the lifetimes we spend throwing the flimsiest threads across the chasm dividing self from self. Of how fiercely we long for human connection, how we yearn and ache to be known. Arthur, on the brink of death, had entrusted me with his story. I was his witness. I knew the truth of him.

'Thank you,' I said. 'Thank you for sharing who you are with me.'

Before I left, I found myself breaking the rules. I wanted to convey the opposite of prejudice. I wanted Arthur to know he was heard, respected, cherished, loved. And so, impulsively, I stretched across the bed. I kissed my patient on his cheek then drew back, to my relief, to see him smiling. He beckoned me closer. I leaned in to the earthiness of illness and fear. Face damp with sweat, shoulders shaking a little, Arthur just managed to kiss my cheek in turn. We were both well aware that his lifetime might be measured in only hours.

Every day, in every hospital, people lie in crumpled cotton beginning to confront the loss of their life. We know what we want our hospitals to be. Places of warmth, safety, kindness and love, particularly for those of us who are frail, fearful, lonely and lost. Places where people are cherished as the unique and precious individuals they are. But, too often, hospitals fall short. Though I have lost count of the thousands of tiny acts of kindness from hospital staff towards their patients, people can still shrink into numbers, diseases, problems, body parts, their stories submerged beneath institutional constraints. They can suffer, unintentionally, at our hands.

I had to make a choice. For a time, haematology was my dream speciality. I loved the nuanced and unpredictable trajectories of blood cancers, the combination of extraordinary cutting-edge science with the highest stakes, life-and-death conversations with patients. I loved, on a good day, being able to save lives. But lodged in the back of my mind remained the night, some years ago now, that I had spent with Dave's mother in her final hours, striving, with my father's help, to ensure she received adequate care. And there were those doctors I still observed in the hospital, curtly dispatching their patients to the 'palliative dustbin' because, apparently, once an illness entered a terminal phase, human lives were no longer deemed worth engaging with.

Despite my love of acute and emergency medicine, I found myself drawn to patients with life-limiting illness precisely, in part, because some other doctors ran a mile. I had seen so many deaths in hospital that were uglier and crueller than they ever should have been. And I knew we should be doing this better.

For all its apparent darkness, palliative medicine, I suspected, might be the one department in the hospital in which I could remain the doctor I had always hoped to be.

8

Light in the Dark

I am terrified by this dark thing
That sleeps in me;
All day I feel its soft, feathery turnings, its
malignity.

Sylvia Plath, 'Elm', *Collected Poems*

It is the kind of scream that stops you dead in your tracks. More howl than human, a torrent of anguish. I find myself sprinting towards the closed door before I have any idea what to do when I enter. Ron, my patient, is mercifully peaceful, but his wife is bent double on the floor.

'Julie,' I murmur, helping her to her feet. 'It's OK. Come on, Julie.'

It is the very furthest thing from OK. She is tossing and writhing in my arms. If any of us, at age eighteen, had married our childhood sweetheart, spent the next forty-odd years in tight-knit matrimony, raised children, adored the grandchildren, and then been forced to look on as the most feared of brain tumours, glioblastoma, remorselessly laid claim to our loved one, we too might find ourselves slumped on hospital linoleum, unable to contain our desperation.

Rarely in my career as a doctor has empathy felt this unwelcome. I do not want to share Julie's feelings – this experience, for her, of gasping for air like a fish on a deck, fighting and flailing to breathe. I want, with every fibre, to stop it.

Ron, serenely, sleeps on. He has no idea where his wife is. The steroids he has been taking to reduce the swelling inside his cranium have redistributed his flesh from his limbs to face and torso. Now his eyes are as sunken beneath swollen cheeks and plumped forehead as his personality is beneath tumour. There are, around his hospice bed, no monitors, no beeping, no lines, no leads, none of the mechanised trappings of modern-day life-saving. Just the fleece blanket from home and a teddy from a grandson, lying askew on the pillow. Ron's oblivion, perhaps, is a blessing. Even as I hold his wife in my arms, trying to comfort and calm her, I note the erratic breathing that can herald death's approach. If he is going – and I think he is, very soon – he is entirely unaware of it.

I have watched Ron deteriorate daily. On Monday, he could smile and squeeze his wife's hand, still able to answer yes and no to his doctor's enquiries. By Tuesday, the words had run dry, but his eyes lit up every time Julie spoke to him. Wednesday brought vacancy. Ron was there but not there, cast adrift, eyes half open, his mind locked away even from the touch of his wife and the voice that had always reached him. On Thursday, he no longer opened his eyes. He breathed deeply, surely, the way a small child sleeps, limbs loose and sprawling, face slack with ease. 'I never thought it would be peaceful,' Julie told me, the irony lost on neither wife nor doctor that, as Ron calmly plumbed greater depths of unconsciousness, the more piercingly dreadful his absence loomed for her.

Now it is Friday. Overnight, Ron has changed unmistakably. Deeply unresponsive, his breathing is fitful. I know, by the faintest whisper of a pulse at his wrist, that his heart is failing rapidly. The mottled colour of his limbs confirms it. His fingertips are cold, his skin grey-tinged as, organ by organ, his body shuts down.

I have been a palliative care doctor for exactly one week. Ron is one of my first hospice patients and, earlier today, I sat with Julie in a quiet room to explain that these were, most likely, her husband's last hours. 'I knew this was coming, I knew it, I knew it,' she muttered distractedly, hands twisting and knotting, as if repeating a phrase could somehow quell the rising sickness in her stomach. The small box of strategically placed NHS tissues looked pitiful, inane in the face of her grief, the pastoral scenes on the walls almost mocking. I resisted the longing to leap for platitudes. No words seemed up to the task. Instead, we sat in silence, her hands held in mine, as the theoretical loss she had known was looming began to take form, in fits and starts, in a tremor, a gasp, her hand clutching her chest as she began to feel the grief burn.

Unlike Julie, I have the luxury of being here by choice. I could flee these four walls, choose a different line of work. Yet if I turned away, left grief's fallout to others, Ron would still be dying, and his wife's heart would still be breaking. And I would be the doctor who had chosen to walk when the act of being present is perhaps, in this moment, the best any physician can offer.

They have been married for forty-six years, longer than I have lived. Old enough to speak of their 'courting' days, Julie has turned the room into a shrine to her husband, a photographic archive of the decades that bind them. There is Ron outside the church, rocking his seventies flares, beaming at his shyly smiling bride. There is a still-teenaged Julie, newborn baby in her arms, its infant hand wrapped tight around its father's outsized thumb. Then, on the window sill, framed portraits of husband, wife and the four children they have raised together fight for space. Next, the retirement cruise snaps – this is a lifetime concertinaed – all cocktails and sunburn and tipsy affection. And, above all, the wall, commandeered in instalments by the visiting grandchildren, now plastered with Blu-tacked affection and tattered sheets of A4. The hand-drawn kittens and unicorns, ragged diggers and aliens, felt-tipped love hearts and stars, and those wiggling, effusive declarations of love – 'Get more well, Granddad.' 'I'm kissing you, Granddad'.

Now, at Ron's bedside, Julie can contain her loss no longer, and its eruption is harsh and terrible. In the old days, doctors used sedatives for moments like this. But were shots of benzodiazepine to stupefy the grief-stricken used to palliate doctors' discomfort first and foremost? I grope for what may actually help, instead of merely obliterate, in this room where conventional medicine no longer has anything to offer. Out of my depth, I blurt out the words: 'Julie, would you like to say goodbye to Ron? I mean, as his wife – would you like to lie next to him?'

The screaming stops. She stares at me, faltering. 'Can – can I do that? Is that even possible?'

I do not know for certain that it is. Ron fills every nook of his specially cushioned bed and I am worried I may cause unintentional harm. But I rally the nurses and together, on their lead, with infinite care, we reposition his inert body. It takes time and skill, but there is just enough space in the bed for Julie to squeeze in beside her husband. She nestles her body against his, holds his hands, strokes his brow, and feels his slow, sighing breaths on her cheek as she tells him over and over, a whispered mantra, that she loves him. I bite my lip and we dim the lights, quietly closing the door behind us on these final, most intimate moments of marriage.

Half an hour or so later, I return to the room just as Ron, still embraced by the woman he first met as a schoolboy, exhales his final breath. So indistinct now is the cusp between his life and its extinction, I can barely discern he has crossed it. A hiatus. A moment of clarity for me, not yet dawned on Julie. Suddenly, mouth agape, she reaches a hand towards me. The gesture, finger-tips splayed and trembling, is a question of such eloquence that words are superfluous. I do not flinch. 'He's gone,' I say, gently but clearly. 'I am so very sorry.'

I am not sure whether anything I have done today was right or appropriate, let alone whether it constituted medicine. In the storm of tears that follows, the nurses hold Julie as she falls apart. Cups of tea, hugs, shoulders to cry on. Diminutive, seemingly inadequate gestures. Yet weeks later, when she returns bearing baskets of gifts for the doctors and nurses, Julie will talk of how much it all meant to her, those acts of kindness from the hospice staff that tempered the time when grief was blinding her.

Three years on from Ron's death, the NHS hospice where I work today is, as then, strikingly beautiful. You would hardly believe we are part of a hospital. Natural light streams in from skylights and floor-to-ceiling French windows, allowing patients to look out on gardens, trees and the birds just outside. There are Jacuzzis, massage, art and music therapy, ice cream and homemade smoothies on tap. For patients who long to take their first proper bath in an age, the nurses have a secret stash of luxury bath bombs. We hold weddings here, set up date nights, sneak in pets, break the rules. There is even a drinks trolley, wheeled from room to room by volunteers twice a day, amply stocked with fine vintages and cans. Because what better way, for those who fancy a drink, of remembering normal life back home?

Bird food and beer might not seem revolutionary, but when I arrived here, seven years after starting life as a doctor, they signalled something thrillingly radical. For all the care and compassion contained within hospital walls, it would be hard to design a more dehumanising space than your typical busy teaching hospital. The desolate architecture of lengthy corridors and neon-lit bays is slave to hygiene and efficiency. Every surface is bare and antiseptically wiped, every light harsh and functional: this is hospital as warehouse of infirm human products.

Indeed, Albert Kahn, a renowned American architect of his day, responsible for some of Ford Motor Company's largest factories, explicitly applied the logic of assembly lines to the spatial organisation of patient care when he designed hospitals such as that of the University of Michigan in 1925. Efficiency, sterility, productivity, spotlessness. Is it any wonder many people want to die at home when the alternative – at the precise moment when sanctity and warmth have, surely, never mattered more – is an environment as soulless as an airport departure gate?

Etymologically speaking, medicine is not what it appears to be. The word 'doctor' originates from the Latin *docere*, meaning 'to teach', while 'patient', from the Latin *patiens*, means 'one who suffers'. The endurance, the quiet stoicism that is required of patients both inside and outside of NHS hospitals never fails to move me – the waiting and waiting for hours in A&E, the languishing on lists, while weeks or even months go by, before starting treatment for cancer, for example. Sometimes too I am struck by the irony that, in inviting our patients to hospital to relieve their suffering, we manage effortlessly to enhance their distress. The gowns, the wristbands, the profound loss of agency as a patient hangs on tenterhooks for what their doctors do next to them. All of it, surely, a form of pain for a species hardwired to act, to decide, to shape, however sketchily, our destiny.

As for both 'hospice' and 'hospital', these words, like 'hospitality', share the same Latin root, *hospes*, meaning 'host', 'guest' or 'stranger'. I like to see my hospice as restoring in some way the bonds of hospitality a hospital fractures, being a kind of hybrid of medicine and domesticity, a halfway house between home and a hospital. The basics of welcoming strangers, offering them food, shelter and safety, can feel like footnotes in the neon expanse of modern hospitals. But in a hospice, art on the walls, plants, colours, textures, views are curated, taken seriously.

For me, walking on to a ward in which aesthetics mattered felt akin to joining a rebel alliance. The hospice space, like its practice, toppled conventional medical paradigms, and from day one my pulse quickened with possibility. Why *can't* a wife curl up in a hospital bed beside her dying husband? Why *can't* we ensure there is a way for an inpatient who knows their precious time is short to have sex with their partner, should they choose to? Why *aren't* we throwing open our doors to teenage children bearing boxes of pizza for movie nights with Dad, before they lose him for ever? *Why* are pet dogs and cats seen as nothing but health hazards when, for comfort, they may surpass anything a human has to offer? And *why* – the most heretical question of all – why are all these questions, and a thousand more like them, not being asked in non-palliative, everyday hospital environments? Why, in short, do you only ever earn a truly patient-centred hospital environment either by being a child, on a children's ward, where surroundings are taken seriously, or by being on the brink of death? Does not every adult human animal deserve this solace in hospital, where distress and anxiety are rife?

One evening, shortly after I join the team, I witness how much environment matters, and how little it can take to transport a patient away from their suffering.

A French accent rings out across the hospice gardens, melodious and clear. 'Excuse me, may I stay here for a moment?' it asks. I hear a rumble of voices – the paramedics, I suspect – and then, to my surprise, laughter, a sound of genuine joy, rising like light from a stretcher.

Adele has spent the last three months of her life in an urban specialist cancer centre. In all that time, she has not felt fresh air. Perhaps she has been too unwell to sit or lie outside, though I suspect her incarceration is accidental, a failure not of Adele's physiology but of her doctors' imagination. When the full might of the medicine machine – the professors, the scientists, a vast and intricate clinical team – is focused single-mindedly on saving life, on a cure, niceties like inviting a patient outside are an afterthought, if considered at all.

Tonight, this young woman, barely thirty years old, has been delivered by ambulance to the hospice to die. I know I will soon be reaching out my hand to hers, and that this first human touch, skin on skin, might do more than any words to welcome her. It is midsummer, a heatwave of such length and intensity that the pale blue dawns, breaking so faithfully, have almost seduced us, a nation of waterlogged stoics, into believing they will last for ever.

Adele has, at most, a few weeks left to live. Fear so often accompanies patients to our doors yet, with late-evening sunshine pouring on to her face, she looks not afraid but exultant. I hear a giggle, a murmur in French I cannot quite catch. Like me, the paramedics are grinning. It could be her beauty, her charm or her Parisian insistence that they wheel her trolley not inside the building but outside, straight into the gardens, yet delightedly they obey. There she basks, eyes closed, face tilted skywards, beaming a smile of pure radiance.

For a moment, unseen, hovering beside the hospice entrance, the doctor in me falters. The word that enters my head is medical blasphemy, but this is nothing less than regeneration. After so many months of being so diminished, pared away piece by piece by her disease, Adele, here and now, is being replenished by nothing so technical as honeysuckle, bees and a blue vault of sky. She is growing while dying, before my eyes.

I know that shortly we will have to talk about tumours. About her second incarceration, of liver, bowel and spleen by her cancer – a cancer so territorially ruthless it has escaped the confines of her body to grow outwards, through her abdominal wall, genetically human yet anatomically monstrous. We will talk about the pain and shame this has unleashed, about whether she is right to care this much, this late, about something as seemingly trivial as bodily form. I will note her fierce determination to apply her make-up in the mornings, when even raising an arm is almost beyond her. Slowly she will come to trust me enough to reveal her fears about how, exactly, death is going to claim her, and whether she will manage to maintain her poise. I will help her write a letter each to her mother and her sister, and birthday cards to nieces not yet three years old. The doors of her bedroom will never be closed, but flung wide to the flowers and skies she loves so deeply. Her smile will continue, if briefly, to outshine the sun.

All this is to come, yet for now I still linger at the hospice doors, startled − as I so often am − by my patients' capacity to savour the present with a passion and intensity that put my casual, half-focused days to shame. Dying from cancer, Adele is incandescent with life, even as her time slips through her fingers like water. Now how does she manage that? Humbled, hopeful, eager to help, I take a step into the sunshine towards her.

Few buildings are steeped in more fear and taboo than a hospice. Patients often see my ward as a precipice, a place where life stories are cruelly cut short. They imagine that, on crossing its threshold, all they will do is plummet downwards, with nothing left to experience but dying. Hope, like life, will be crushed.

Recently, I met a new patient for the first time, a Star Wars fan with end-stage heart failure. As he arrived on the ward he said, somewhat ruefully, 'I've always thought of this place as the Death

Star.' I could see how much the effort at lightness cost him. 'Well,' I smiled, taking his lead, 'let me try and aim more for Princess Leia than Darth Vader.' He managed a grin in return – the tentative start, I hoped, of a therapeutic relationship – but, for now, his fear was palpable, as though the act of arrival had sealed his fate, sentenced him to imminent extinction.

I too first set foot here with dread. Multiple times, in fact. A very junior doctor at the time, I used to be responsible, during my nights on-call, for patients across the entire hospital site including, to my intense unease, those tucked away in the hospice. Even at the best of times, night shifts in a sprawling hospital necessitated miles of traipsing through empty corridors. But the hospice was right on the site's periphery. To reach it, you had to exit the main building and scuttle, alone, across deserted car parks and derelict scrub in the darkness. I always shivered at my own vulnerability, distinctly aware that, were something catastrophic to happen in the shadows, no one would locate my body until morning.

On finally reaching the hospice, the ubiquity of dying unnerved me. If doctors cannot fix things, then what is the point of us? What words could I find for these patients to comfort them? Should I confront or skirt the topic of death? Would their decaying bodies, so close to extinction, be too much for me? How on earth did palliative care doctors surround themselves, day in, day out, with all this misery yet still, inexplicably, come out smiling? Churning inside, I would creep on to the ward, secretly hoping for a nice, straightforward crash call to whisk me away from this benighted place, both literally and metaphorically cloaked in darkness.

In fact, of course, the hospice patients I encountered at night were not some alien breed, rendered otherworldly by their proximity to death. They were simply patients, people, just like all of us. Sometimes afraid, sometimes in pain, sometimes delighted to chat to a doctor in the long and lonely small hours. My nocturnal trepidation was inspired not by what was *actually* there, in the hospice, but by what I thought, or feared, was lurking. My imagination, not mortality, was the fundamental problem – the lurid properties with which my mind had invested death. I had attributed qualities of awfulness to dying patients that they did not intrinsically possess.

Nevertheless, my fears persisted. Even after resolving to specialise in palliative medicine, the decision was less a conviction than a leap of faith. Indeed, during my early days in the hospice I felt like a brand-new doctor all over again, learning an alternative medical paradigm, one with people, not diseases, at its heart.

'Right, I've got a plan, everyone. Entonox. Seriously. If it works for giving birth, it'll work for this too.'

I scanned the room, intrigued by other people's reactions. The chaplain looked alarmed, the social worker raised an eyebrow. The notion of laughing gas, nitrous oxide, as a means of facilitating labour was one thing, but *dying*? Was this really advisable? I could see the other doctors in the room visibly struggling to wrap their heads around it.

Nina, the nurse who had made the suggestion, laughed, enjoying our consternation. One of the most experienced nurses in the hospice, her sheer warmth and ebullience had an uncanny knack of reaching even the most distressed of patients. She possessed the rare ability, on entering a patient's room, to bring in a touch of lightness too, as though the world, no matter how dark, had just become a sweeter, safer place to be.

'You know, I think she might be on to something,' agreed Laurie, our ward sister, the heart and soul of the hospice.

We were sitting in the weekly 'MDT', a multidisciplinary team meeting in which everyone – doctors, nurses, physiotherapists, occupational therapists, chaplains and social workers – comes together to discuss in great depth each patient's needs. Many medical specialities pay lip service to teamwork – the doctors, invariably, calling the shots – but this, I could see, was the real thing. Everyone present was currently vexed by the challenge of how to help an exceptionally frail patient in her late eighties, admitted with an aggressive cancer that had caused multiple fractures to her bones.

Too weak to withstand surgery to fix these, Florence was forced instead to endure the grate of bone on splintered bone. She lay rigid in bed, too scared to move, waiting for pain to ambush her. Yet her leanness – she was scarcely more than a skeleton wrapped in parchment – meant the nurses had to do the one thing she dreaded: reposition her in bed, every few hours, to protect her from developing damage to her paper skin. No matter how gently they did so, no matter how much morphine we used, nothing could assuage Florence's terror of the agony she was certain was about to come.

Somehow – and I would swiftly discover she made a habit of creative compassion – Nina had intuited exactly what might help. Entonox sees multiple women through the suffering of childbirth not primarily by suppressing the pain, but by enabling them to cease to care about it. Fast-acting and potent – part fairy dust, part Jägerbomb – the drug blots away the cares of the world. If anything could quash Florence's anticipatory terror, Entonox might be it.

'I'm going to try it tonight,' Nina announced. 'Florence loves music. We'll have a little Entonox party.'

I grinned. It was impossible not to. This, my first hospice MDT, felt a little like the Wild West of medicine. Partying after dark with laughing gas and morphine? Not exactly a textbook approach to pain management. But Nina's logic, I could see, was impeccable. Neurobiological research shows that our perception of pain is highly dependent on the context in which it occurs and can bear little relationship to the extent of any wounds. There are reports of soldiers in battle, for example, who have suffered multiple fractures of the largest bones in their body, yet describe only twinges of pain. Focusing one's full attention on pain is known to exacerbate it, while distraction can be highly effective in reducing patients' pain. It has been shown, for instance, that severe burns patients undergoing treatments or physiotherapy report only a fraction of their pain when distracted with a virtual-reality-style video game during the procedure.

Nina had a smile that could light up Manhattan. Virtual reality had nothing on her. I left work full of hope she would crack this and, the next morning, rushed to find her.

'Nina, what happened with Florence? How did it go? Did it work?'

'Did it work? Rach, it was bloody fantastic. I put on Gloria Gaynor, we were both singing our guts out. The Entonox was brilliant and, you know what? She hardly even noticed when we moved her. It worked like a dream.'

'Ha! Nina, that is amazing. You are amazing. I can honestly

say, in the nicest possible way, there is no one I'd rather have at my deathbed than you.'

Laughing and humming, Nina swept away down the ward, a one-woman force for good.

Later, when I went to see Florence myself, her face lit up as she described her evening visit from Nina. Briefly, the cumulative assaults of cancer fell away. 'I do love listening to my daughters' disco music,' she mused, almost sheepishly. 'I just forgot to be worried. And then it didn't hurt like before. And I realised it might not hurt like that next time.' Suddenly, she giggled. From deep within the folds of time, there might even have been a glimpse of the schoolgirl she had been so many years ago. I saw, in an instant, that what Nina had restored was perhaps the most vital of all qualities in hospital. She had given her patient hope.

Similar plot-twisting acts of attentiveness are ubiquitous in my hospice. When the staff knock up a fresh smoothie from blackberries and bananas, its preparation tells a tale of how much its recipient matters. When the massage therapist takes a patient's palms and kneads a little stress away, her fingertips speak of indulgence and gratification. You are worth it, you are worth it, you are worth it.

Perhaps the heaviest moments I experience at work are those when a patient, invariably elderly, confesses their belief that terminal illness has reduced them to nothing, a nobody, a waste of space that only burdens their loved ones. Death's imminence stains their final days with a terrible, inescapable pointlessness. But the story they tell themselves is bogus. Its opposite is true. Every one of us is dying from the first intake of breath, the clock remorselessly ticking down. So either all our days are futile, or every one counts, perhaps none more so than the last. As the founder of the palliative care movement, the British nurse-turned-physician Dame Ciccly Saunders, once wrote: 'You matter because you are you, and you matter to the end of your life. We will do all we can not only to help you die peacefully, but also to live until you die.'

For Florence, my patient whose fear of future pain blighted so terribly her present, her dread, I suspected, stemmed in part from what her pain represented. As if severe pain is not bad enough, imagine experiencing every spasm as a klaxon of doom, a megaphone roar from a body declaring its own annihilation. Small wonder the anticipation of pain is unbearable if, in your mind, pain and death are synonymous.

In palliative medicine, perhaps more than in any other speciality, the stories we tell ourselves have devastating potency. Dying, a once-in-a-lifetime experience, is never known first hand until the moment of extinction. In the absence of familiarity, in the space of the unknown, our worst fears can thrive. What we call death is therefore a marriage of the physical fact of our finitude with the roving, unbounded human imagination. The dark stories we may conjure about our end – that it will be intolerably painful, undignified, lonely or grim – can never be debunked by science, not least because the narratives themselves help construct the endings. At the end of life, as Florence experienced, fearing the worst may increase its chances of happening.

In navigating this complex web of fact, fear, imagination and physiology, a palliative care doctor is a scientist with a hint of shaman. The importance of hard, evidence-based medicine – the savviest pharmacology, the best diagnostic acumen, the ability to appraise with ruthless objectivity the pros and cons of various treatment options – goes without saying. But it only gets you so far. When your patients are confronting not merely a constellation of symptoms but their existential anguish at their own extermination, the role of doctor can encompass that of counsellor, teacher, parent and priest.

Contrary to many people's fears, patients do not, typically, arrive at a hospice to die. Usually, only a small proportion of a hospice's work centres around their inpatient beds. There will, in addition, be huge amounts of day centre and community activity. Patients who are well enough to travel to and from the hospice – usually at an earlier stage in their illness – may attend their day centre for months, even years. Simultaneously, hospice nurses and doctors extend their reach outwards, into people's own homes, care homes and all the other parts of a hospital, providing care and expertise to patients, families and non-specialist medical teams. Even in the inpatient hospice setting – where only patients with the most complex symptoms such as severe pain, nausea, breathlessness and agitation tend to be seen – patients often become well enough to be discharged home after a brief hospice stay.

Our day centre crackles with life. Alongside an art and music therapist, patients may choose to write songs, paint watercolours, play the piano, sing. They often forge intense friendships, supporting and encouraging each other. The food is good, the laughter loud. Once, on arriving at work one Easter Sunday, I found our staff room filled with chocolate nests containing sugar mini eggs, prepared with love the day before – an act of kindness from the day-centre patients towards the hospice staff. I was reminded, yet again, that a terminal diagnosis is not a sentence, but the beginning of a process that may take years to unfold, containing love, hope, generosity and kindness, alongside the inevitable sorrow and loss. It is, in short, a part of life, the urgent business of being human.

'Death doesn't feel like it's coming,' said one of my patients. 'I still feel full of life.' Theresa, a tiny woman in her sixties, sharp and bright as a wren, had been diagnosed with an autoimmune disease, systemic sclerosis, which had been kept at bay for many years by immunosuppressants. Recently, the drugs had begun to stop working and her kidneys and lungs were now failing. She knew she was probably in her last year of life, but when she received a phone call from the hospice inviting her to visit the day centre, her first thought was, 'What are they not telling me? If I go there I might never come out.'

Theresa inhabited a disorientating hinterland, neither entirely healthy nor overwhelmingly ill. 'I knew what was looming, I just didn't think it belonged to me yet. "Where am I?" I remember thinking. "Am I still living or have I started dying?"'

Dislocated, her sense of self shredded by her illness, she decided, in the spirit of adventure, to give the day centre a go. To her surprise, on arrival, encouraged by the music therapist, she found herself picking up a pen. 'It must have been fifty years since I last wrote a poem. I'd have been a schoolgirl, forced to do it in English lessons. Never written poetry since.' The poems began to pour out of her. Inspired by everyday moments she loved – watching a robin eating worms on the lawn outside her kitchen, sitting in the sunshine with her grandson and his ball – she found herself preserving the flow of her life in pages of verse.

'I don't think I am consciously trying to stop time. I just love it all so much,' Theresa told me, smiling sadly. 'I notice moments I might not have noticed before. Everything inspires me to write.'

Rather than succumbing to fatalistic despair, it seemed that Theresa had been galvanised, energised by her curtailed life expectancy. I asked her whether, for her, death was a catalyst.

'I think I just appreciate the sheer pleasure of being alive. We forget how very beautiful the world is, don't we?'

Later that day, I thought about time and transience, about the loveliness of living things, about the fact that we are all destined to die. And I thanked my lucky stars I worked here in the Death Star, among the men and women who showed me how to live.

9

A Piece of Work

I can't go on. I'll go on.

Samuel Beckett, *The Unnamable*

'Please let me know the moment he arrives,' I said to Nina as soon as I'd heard the patient's story. Simon was a man in extremis. Blue-lighted from home, and on his way to the hospice, he had a cancer of his thyroid that was threatening to suffocate him. Already requiring oxygen at home, this morning his breathing had taken a turn for the worse and now, we had been told, he was fighting for air.

Simon, a former policeman in his sixties, had retired a few months earlier. He was looking forward to having time to while away in the fresh air, walking and jogging. Shortly afterwards, he had noticed a lump in his neck, painless, innocuous and perhaps, he had assumed, related to a recent head cold. But the lump, unlike the cold, persisted and, more unnervingly, continued to grow. Still more curious than concerned – he regularly ran ten miles before breakfast – Simon visited his GP.

The speed of his referral to hospital impressed him, innocent of the fact that he was on a two-week cancer pathway, its celerity commensurate with his doctor's worst fears. There was to be no well-earned peace in the countryside for Simon. The scan became a biopsy, and the biopsy a consultant, murmuring cryptically about inoperability, as Simon sat stricken, pinned to his seat, hearing nothing of substance after 'cancer'.

I heard him before I set eyes on him. Specifically, I heard the sound of air being sucked into his lungs through an airway severely compressed by tumour. Stridor – the harsh rasp of air with each intake of breath, audible only when the trachea is critically narrowed. Once heard, never forgotten. Patients with stridor have nowhere to go. If the obstruction worsens, they will suffocate.

When I entered his room, Simon was sitting bolt upright, eyes darting frantically, his shirt ripped off and both hands gripping the bed like his life depended on it. From deep inside his body, from the depths of his spinal cord, he trembled with fear. Beside him stood a woman in her thirties, distraught and dishevelled, saying, 'It's OK, Dad. Look. Look, the doctor's here. Everything's going to be OK now.'

Simon stared up at me, beads of sweat on his brow, gulping for air. There was no way he could sustain this work of breathing. At the same time, I observed, the oxygen required to keep his saturations healthy was sufficiently low to be delivered not through a mask, but through small tubes in the nose. Although petrified, and with good reason, he was not – yet – in respiratory failure.

In an A&E department, Simon would have been whipped straight to Resus, gowned, cannulated and hooked up to lines and monitoring, all within moments of arrival. I chose instead, you might argue, to gamble. If Simon was about to die, I reasoned, none of this paraphernalia was going to prevent that. But if, as I suspected, panic had exacerbated his airway obstruction, then I knew how to help.

I ascertained from Sophie, Simon's daughter, that he had completed radiotherapy to his thyroid a few days earlier. His oncologist's hope had been to shrink the tumour, eking out a little more time, perhaps even enabling him to reach his grandson's sixth birthday. It was not much of a hope, but it was something.

'Simon, I am confident we can help you feel better,' I began, 'but before we talk properly, I'd like to be quick and efficient, examining you, sorting out some treatment straight away. Then we can talk. Is that OK?'

He nodded, mute, every sinew in his neck and chest straining to drag air into his lungs.

I worked fast. The nurses brought the large dose of steroids that would, I hoped, begin to shrink the swelling in Simon's neck. Next, a tiny dose of a fast-acting sedative, just enough to take the edge off his panic.

'Would you like me to explain what I think is happening?' I asked him, keen to allow the sedative a little more time to calm his fears.

'Yes,' he said clearly – the first word he had been capable of speaking out loud.

I spoke evenly, unhurriedly, hoping to instil trust and confidence. 'I think there are two problems, Simon. First, there is your tumour, pressing on your windpipe, but there is also the radiotherapy, which has damaged the tissues in your throat and caused them to swell. We see this very commonly, we're used to looking after it. The breathing often becomes worse for a few days after radiotherapy, maybe a week or so, before it gets better. Steroids can really help bring down the swelling.'

As I talked, Simon's eyes never left me. His gasps, I noticed, were beginning to decelerate.

'How does it feel now? Is the injection we just gave you helping at all?'

'Well, I don't feel quite as bad,' he said doubtfully.

Out of the corner of my eye I saw that Sophie, positioned just out of her father's line of sight, was crying.

'Simon, I'd like to try something. I think we can turn down your oxygen a little. You're managing 100 per cent saturations now. I think you might not even need so much of it.'

Reluctantly, he allowed me to do so, and began to describe living alone with his cancer, having been widowed a few years previously. 'It's all been so quick. Too much to take in. Sophie, if I'm honest, is my rock, but she has Timmy, her boy, to look after as well.'

'Don't be ridiculous, Dad,' Sophie interjected, almost angrily. 'You know looking after you is no problem. We all love being with you, especially Timmy.'

Simon could not meet his daughter's eye. His chest, damp with sweat, still undulated with muscle, a torso sculpted from lifelong activity, not yet effaced by cancer. A tattooed tiger stalked up his forearm. Another, imprinted on his shoulder, simply read 'Love'. I wondered how much it cost him to appear this vulnerable in his daughter's eyes, and whether shame was inflaming his distress.

Gently, I kept tweaking the oxygen downwards. 'Simon, you

know this is really encouraging? You're managing to talk in full sentences. I dropped the oxygen down as low as it will go a good ten minutes ago. May I try taking it off you?'

'You're a sly one,' he exclaimed, with the faintest hint of a smile.

'Yep,' I replied with a grin. 'Thoroughly devious, we doctors.'

Tentatively, the hint of a relationship forged, I broached the topic of the future.

He cut me off instantly. 'Look, I'm not stupid,' he exclaimed. 'I don't have one, do I? This is it. I know what's going on.'

'Dad,' pleaded Sophie, tears flowing. 'She's trying to help. Don't shout at her.'

There are moments in medicine when what you say next feels as pregnant with risk as a surgeon's first incision. The right words, used wisely, can bridge the airiest expanse between you and your patient but, if misjudged, may blow trust to pieces. In scarcely a month, cancer had snatched from this man of action and authority his health, his future, his strength and his fear-lessness. And today, perhaps worse than all of that, his daughter had witnessed him writhing in fear, stripped of all composure by the conviction he was dying.

So the words I uttered next were critical. Few sensations are more terrifying than that of fighting to breathe against an obstructed airway. In that moment, every mental sinew you have ever possessed – lifelong habits of logic, love, faith and reason – are wiped out by a frenzied craving for air. The only thing that matters in life is oxygen. Everything else is mere flotsam. Simon had been fighting for his life, the most power-ful and desperate of all human instincts. I needed to give him control, if only over our conversation.

'Simon, are you the kind of person who likes to discuss everything frankly,' I began, 'or do you prefer to take things one day at a time, without speculating about the future?'

'I already know I'm dying,' he responded. 'What else could you possibly tell me?'

'Well, people often assume that once you arrive here, you will never leave. But around half of our patients don't die here. They go home again once we've managed to sort out their symptoms. It's not always a one-way ticket.'

He blinked. No one said anything for a while, as we listened uncomfortably to the scrape of his stridor. Finally, it was his daughter who spoke: 'I didn't realise that, Dad. Did you?'

Silence. My intuition was that Simon not only feared never leaving the hospice, but was also convinced he was imminently dying. Perhaps the only way to reach him was to confront this head on.

'One of the things I've noticed working here, Simon, is how often patients feel unable to ask about the thing they're most preoccupied with, which is what it's actually going to be like when they die – and I wonder whether this is something you'd like to talk about?'

I saw a flash of horror distort Sophie's face, as though I'd trespassed somewhere no doctor should tread; but her father, if anything, looked relieved. 'Go on,' he said cautiously, giving nothing away.

'OK. But please stop me at any point if you don't want me to continue.'

I glanced at Sophie. Simon confirmed that he wanted her to stay.

'So ... we tend to see the same patterns over and over

in people with cancer, or another terminal illness, who are approaching the end of life. Even though the specific diseases are different, the end is often surprisingly similar. One of the first things many patients notice is losing their strength, their energy. Things they used to take in their stride become a real physical and mental effort. I'm guessing you're already aware of that?'

A rueful roll of the eyes. 'No kidding. I used to run marathons. Can't even get up the stairs now.'

'That loss of energy gradually worsens. You might find you need a nap most days, more than one, probably. Then, one day, you realise you're sleeping more than you're awake. It's not painful or horrible, it's just immensely frustrating. Patients can find it helps to try and plan in advance a bit, saving up their energy for the things that really matter.'

'Like Timmy,' Simon interrupted. 'I like to know when he's visiting so I can have a sleep beforehand.'

'I didn't realise that, Dad,' said Sophie.

'Well, I want to give him my best, don't I? And I don't want to lose a second with him.'

Sophie now turned to me. 'Timmy's dad's not around any more, you see. Left when he was two. Only shows up around Christmas and birthdays. Dad's more like his real father.'

'I see,' I said slowly, computing the layers of loss, more intricate and heftier than I ever imagined.

By now, I noted, Simon had been breathing calmly for half an hour without requiring any additional oxygen. Encouraged, I went on.

'Often, at the end, there aren't any dramatic changes. That sleepiness continues. A patient finds they are sleeping nearly all of the time. You stop feeling hungry and you don't want to eat. You may stop feeling thirsty too. Then, one day, rather than sleeping, you slip into unconsciousness. It's not a distinction you are even aware of. Your brain is just more deeply unresponsive. Sometimes, I wonder if this is the body's way of protecting the mind – you stop being afraid, you're oblivious to it all.'

I paused, trying to gauge Simon's reaction. It crossed my mind that whatever form of policing he had done, he must have excelled at inscrutability. No response.

'Shall I go on?' I asked.

The most perfunctory of nods, so I continued.

'You might be thinking that what you've experienced today is nothing like what I've just described. You've felt as though you're suffocating to death and I can't imagine how awful that must be. But what I can promise you is that, if you feel like that again, and even if there is nothing we can do to fix your breathing, we will still be able to help you. We can take away that feeling of panic with drugs that work almost instantly. The injection, the midazolam you had a little while ago can make someone who's crawling the walls not care about anything. I gave you the tiniest dose we can possibly give – a smidge of the stuff. You don't need to feel like that again. We will be right here for you, whatever happens.'

Both Simon and Sophie were quietly crying. The sky was darkening outside. We were sitting, I realised, in a small pool of light from the adjustable lamp just above Simon's bed. A father, a daughter and a doctor, surrounded by shadow, staring together at the death to come. Weighing it, considering its shape and form, perhaps for the very first time. The hostility with which Simon had been bristling was gone.

'How long do you think I have left?' he asked me directly.

'I have no reason to think you are going to die today, Simon. I'm not even certain the blockage in your airway is what will kill you. You might end up getting steadily sleepier, just like I described. I think the radiotherapy has made things worse before making things better, and I'm hoping that starting the steroids will get you through the next few days, dampening down the swelling. Then, all being well, we'll find the radiotherapy will have done its job of shrinking back your tumour. I do think your time is short – weeks, not months, perhaps only very short weeks – but I would love to believe we can get you home for a bit, if that's what you would like. Of course, if you feel safer staying here, that's no problem either. You're the boss, you tell us what you want. Why don't you see how you go over the next day or so? No rush. Just take things a day at a time.'

For a while, Simon said nothing. The silence, though thick with emotion, was not strained. Finally, he raised his eyes to mine and smiled. 'OK. I will. Maybe I'll get to my boy's birthday too. Thank you, Rachel – I mean it.'

My heart, for a beat, threatened to knock me off balance but only later, that night, did I allow myself to feel. A dying man had looked his end in the eye – all of it, the worst of it, potential suffocation – and yet, in that moment of profound mortal reckoning, with every single thing he loved quivering and wilting and slipping from his grasp, had found within himself the strength to look outwards, towards what mattered more than anything: the human beings he loved. How, I wondered, could someone be so aghast at their weakness while behaving with such unseen strength?

I cried that night. But not for what we lose. It is who we

are – our fearful, indomitable, turbulent hearts – that moves me, time and again, in the hospice. When people ask me if my job is depressing, I reply that nothing could be further from the truth. All that is good in human nature – courage, compassion, our capacity to love – is here in its most distilled form. So often, so reliably, I witness people rising to their best, upon facing the worst. I am surrounded by human beings at their finest. Shakespeare's Hamlet, the cynic, may have meant it with bitterness, but I whisper it with awe at work: 'What a piece of work is a man.'

From our earliest moments, we are taught to flinch from death. When the pet guinea pig dies and we sob inconsolably, our parents, desperate to make things better, reach for sugar-coating and denial: 'It's all right, darling, he's gone up to heaven. Yes, he'll still be able to eat beetroot there. Yes, I do know it's his favourite.'

My alternative hot take on death, during the rodent-owning phase of childhood, was encapsulated in the fate of poor Speedy Gonzales. One gerbil, three devoted small children, a sugar-free parable of real-life dying. First, Speedy's racing days were cruelly cut short when my sister accidentally dropped him. Then, Dad took one look at him dragging his broken body across the kitchen floor, legs trailing uselessly behind him, and whisked him off for some emergency medicine.

'What are you going to do?' I whispered.

'His back's broken, Rachel. He needs chloroform.'

As Dad committed covert rodent euthanasia in the upstairs bathroom, we enthusiastically excavated a gerbil-sized grave beneath the apple tree outside. Mum found an empty box of kitchen matches which, when lined with cotton wool, made a perfect, if snug, coffin. But, by the time we were ready for Speedy to be interred, the laws of biochemistry had taken hold. Rigor mortis had turned the gerbil to stone. And the coffin, it turned out, was several sizes too small. We watched, aghast, as Dad rammed rigid rodent against cardboard, muttering under his breath, 'I can't get the bloody thing in.'

'Dad!' we howled, outraged by this sacrilege.

'Mark!' shouted Mum, equally disapproving.

'It's just a gerbil,' he insisted, 'and it's dead.'

In the garden until bedtime, we played at being in mourning. Speedy's freshly dug grave was adorned with apple blossom. We decorated our homemade wooden crucifixes with felt-tipped hearts. It was easily as much fun as an episode of *Tarzan* – the ceremony, the eulogies, the secret shared hope that, if we grieved particularly vocally, we might increase our chances of future pet gerbils being upgraded to hamsters.

The temptation to assure someone, dishonestly, that everything will be all right is as hard to resist on a ward as it is in a playroom. What doctor does not ache to take away the fear with words? To defer their patient's grief with tenuous promises and magical thinking? I would dearly love to claim that, with good palliative care, no one ever suffers when they die. Were I to do so, of course, I would be propagating a lie. The losses that mount during a terminal illness – of function, of form, of independence, of self-control – can be so terribly hard to bear, for example, and are beyond the reach of doctors. But the one thing I can assert with confidence, based on the thousands of patients for whom I have cared, is that rarely, in a hospice, do people's fears of the manner in which they will die match the lived reality.

Simon is a case in point. Few modes of dying are as dreadful as that of suffocation. We will open an extra bed, pull out all the stops, to bring someone into the hospice at risk of airway obstruction. But once here, even with symptoms as desperate as Simon's, modern palliative drugs are a match for almost anything.

The morning after he arrived, I went to see Simon on my ward round. Even before entering his room, I knew he was better. The most ominous rasp in the world, that of stridor, was gone. I walked in to see him eating Weetabix for breakfast.

'Well . . . hello,' I grinned, delighted. He put down his spoon. 'This I did not expect to see. Simon, how are you feeling?'

'Honestly? Like a new man. Those steroids must have done their stuff, right?'

Indeed they had. In suppressing the swelling of damaged tissues in his neck, they had given Simon back his airway.

'I've been thinking about what you said yesterday,' he told me. 'I'd like to get home for a bit, if I can. But then I'd like to come here, when things get worse again, because I feel safe here. I know I'll be looked after.'

Over the next few days, liberated from the terror of fighting for air, Simon managed to enjoy sitting out in the hospice gardens. Then, one day, I entered his room to find a mopheaded ruffian curled up in his arms, happily chomping his way through the Quality Street. Sophie sat quietly in the corner.

'Granddad can't play with me like he used to,' announced Timmy, as though we were mid-conversation, 'because he's too poorly.'

'Is that right?' I replied. 'But I bet he still gives awesome cuddles, doesn't he?'

Timmy squirmed around to face his surrogate dad, half gig-gling, half hiding with bashfulness.

'Oh yes, he does,' said Simon to the wriggling polecat in his lap. 'The best tickles too, if you're not careful, Timmy.'

In the spirit of unvarnished honesty – no sugar-coating, not even for stridor – I confess that Simon never achieved his wish of returning home. The steroids worked wonders in helping his breathing but, after a week of optimism, he started to tire. The cancer of his thyroid was particularly virulent and had begun to overwhelm him.

'Do you think he'll make it to Timmy's birthday?' Sophie asked me in the corridor.

'I'm afraid I'm doubtful,' I answered truthfully. Timmy was due to turn six in a week or so's time, but Simon was deteri-orating daily. 'I have an idea, though. Would Timmy mind if perhaps you brought his birthday forward this year?'

A few days later, balloons were taped to the outside of Simon's door. A sign read 'Timmy's Birthday Party'. When he saw it, he squealed with delight, racing inside to fling his arms around Granddad. The fury of unwrapping, paper flying everywhere, family and friends sipping Prosecco around the bedside. A toy light sabre, a teddy, a birthday cake in the shape of Buzz Lightyear, the singing, the laughter, the painful haggardness of the man in the centre of it all, whose eyes nonetheless seemed to glow.

The next morning, when I arrived at work, Simon was unrousable. He died two days later, his daughter at his side, without ever regaining consciousness. There was, in the end, no panic or fighting or flailing to breathe, just the ebbing of life like a tide in retreat, quietly unveiling cold sand.

*

Patients, understandably, do not typically arrive at a hospice with an open mind. Usually, like Simon, they have a pre-drafted script for what is going to happen to them. It involves suffering, pain and surrender to others. Sometimes, a patient may be so terrified of entering the ward that they flinch from their bed as though it is the cold, damp earth of their grave. Friends and family members can be equally tormented. We will use morphine, they may worry, to hasten their loved one's demise. Syringe drivers, in particular, are feared as tools of mercy killing. Neither is true — indeed, both would be criminal — but these suspicions, invariably, are kept under wraps unless gently coaxed out into the open.

I therefore meet each new patient assuming everything and nothing. All and none of these narratives may apply. I hope that with time, respect, patience and attentiveness, my patients may come to reveal what burdens them. I know that our greatest challenge is often not the management of complex symptoms but, rather, giving someone the belief that they can rewrite their script.

On one occasion, the script had remarkable precision. Dorothy was admitted to the hospice on a Monday. 'There is no point in spending time with me,' she declared on arrival. 'I will be dead on Thursday.'

'What makes you think that?' I asked, intrigued.

She gave me the kind of lingering stare a teacher reserves for the classroom dunce. Then, with surprising vigour, explained: 'Mr Edwards. I take it you do know who Mr Edwards is? The senior consultant on the surgical ward. Did he not communicate this with you? He told me my bowels had stopped working and I would be dead in six days. And that was on Friday. I have three days left.'

I knew the rudiments of Dorothy's story. Admitted to A&E with acute bowel obstruction, the cause of which was unclear. But given her age – ninety-six – an almost certainly terminal diagnosis. A transfer to the hospice was arranged. But at no stage in the notes was there mention of Thursday.

'I will concede I do not feel full of death,' Dorothy stated. 'I feel full of life, quite frankly. But if you don't mind, I would rather be left alone now. I have very little time left and I would like to read my newspaper.'

Rarely in my career had I been dismissed more magnificently. I hardly dared to respond. 'I promise to leave in just a moment,' I told Dorothy, 'but I do think it's important to mention that sometimes, even when what will happen next has seemed crystal clear, a person's circumstances change. Based on my medical assessment today, I am not at all certain you will be dead on Thursday. If you had more time, is there any way in particular you would like to spend it?'

Again, that piercing stare, more impatient this time. 'Were I not to be dead on Thursday, then I would certainly be playing bridge with my local group, as I have done every Thursday for the last two decades. But I can assure you I will be dying instead.'

'How about this,' I proposed, as a compromise. 'We plan for bridge, unless death intervenes? Would you like me to see if I can organise to get you there?'

'Young lady, I will humour you if it makes you feel useful.' And with that, she picked up her copy of *The Times*.

'Thank you,' I smiled, to the sports page. 'I'll see what I can do.'

*

The Latin verb *palliare*, meaning 'to cloak', implies that the primary aim of palliative medicine is to disguise and suppress the symptoms of dying, as though the best you can hope for, as death draws near, is to benumb your pain with a morphine haze. But we can do better than that. If a single principle underpins palliative care, it is that living and dying are not binary opposites. The dying, as Dorothy proved so splendidly, are still very much alive.

A good day, for me, in the hospice, is undeniably one in which I feel we have helped someone die with comfort and dignity intact. But infinitely preferable are the days when we have helped a dying patient *live* – be that through sharing a meal with friends in a family area, watching a movie in bed with the kids, basking in a bath filled with insanely priced bubblebath, stroking the family Labrador as he tries to eat the chocolates, saying a rushed but no less momentous 'I do' from a wheelchair decked in flowers in the hospice chapel, or watching goldfinches gleam in the trees outside. No need for flashiness or fanfares, drumrolls and gasps. In a ward where every patient has a terminal diagnosis, life, in all its loveliness, goes on.

I have a partner in crime in the hospice. Jenny takes the fundamental aim of occupational therapy – helping patients achieve their maximum independence in the activities that matter to them – and turns it into a ninja art form. Over and over I have watched her bring patients from a place of suffering to an experience they never believed was possible. Tiny, ebullient and obsessed with otters, she does not so much save life as conjure it. And I knew she was going to love Dorothy.

'What do you reckon then?' I asked Jenny on Tuesday. 'Death or bridge on Thursday?'

She burst out laughing, before describing in detail how Dorothy had summarily dismissed her. Jenny and I like to codename our plots. Because we knew nothing about bridge, and had only the vaguest notion that playing cards were involved, we misnamed this one 'Operation Royal Flush'. I learned only later that this is a winning hand in poker and, besides, the regal connotations befitted the subject. By Wednesday, with characteristic focus and zeal, Jenny had a wheelchair taxi booked to take Dorothy to the village bridge club, various blue-rinsed bridge partners on standby to call us in case of emergency, and a niece coming in that afternoon to deliver Dorothy's all-important pearls and twinset. 'The olive green,' she had instructed us.

On Thursday morning, the nurses barred anyone from entering Dorothy's room as they busied themselves with washing, sprucing, plumping and preening. When she finally emerged, ninety-six years old and still a force to be reckoned with, she could have been Boudica. Desperately thin, her chariot a wheelchair, a pre-emptive dose of morphine in her veins, yet nonetheless sitting ramrod straight with crocodile handbag perched on her lap and an impeccably coordinated green tweed skirt, cashmere cardigan and court shoes. Flushed with all the fuss and attention, Dorothy was, for that Thursday only, the queen of our ward – and she knew it.

For a moment, our eyes met, and she nodded imperceptibly. Not quite a thank you and certainly not an acknowledgement that I had been right – I suspected such a thing happened perhaps once a decade – but more, I felt, a shared understanding that here, indeed, was something to relish, a guerrilla raid to snatch back a speck of stolen future, a chance to live while dying.

The next morning, when I arrived at her bedside to hear all about her trip to the bridge club, Dorothy bemoaned her poor form. 'I simply wasn't as sharp as usual,' she lamented.

I raised an eyebrow. 'To be fair, Dorothy, no one else around the table had the excuse that they were dying,' I observed. 'Did anyone else seem to mind?'

A mischievous grin, a twinkle in her eye, and then, finally, I was liberated from the dunce's corner with the words: 'Dr Clarke, it was magnificent.'

A few days later, Dorothy died. Mr Edwards, it turned out, was wrong by only forty-eight hours, but in that time, how his patient lived. It should not have taken working in a hospice to teach me that for all the fragility of human existence – our lives impossibly brief against the weight of world and time – life is life is life. There is always a spark of beauty or significance to be found in the life you have left, even – perhaps especially – at its end.

Shortly after I started work in my hospice, the poet Helen Dunmore was nearing the last stages of a terminal illness. Her final collection of poetry, *Inside the Wave*, has as its central subject mortality, seen through the prism of her experience of cancer. To be alive, the note on the reverse cover of the book tells us, 'is to be inside the wave, always travelling until it breaks and is gone'. Dunmore was writing beneath that crest, on the brink of toppling and crashing down, conscious that the waves would keep on breaking long after she died. None of this stopped her finding an almost luminous beauty in the world around her, noticing, for example, while lying on an operating table, a therapeutic installation – a waterfall – positioned just outside the theatre doors. She describes her sudden 'amazement and joy' at this indoor cataract, rejoicing at finding her favourite element, water, so unexpectedly near, even as the theatre staff strolled indifferently past.

Seven months after she died, aged sixty-four, Dunmore received the posthumous honour of being awarded the 2017 Costa Book Prize. The next morning, I listened transfixed to her daughter, Tess Charnley, speaking on BBC Radio 4's *Today* programme about how her mother had helped her confront her fears of dying. 'I suppose because I'm quite young, maybe naive, I've always seen death as something very frightening,' said Tess. 'My mum just showed me that it doesn't have to be. I think although her world got smaller, she couldn't go out so far afield, she continued to just see the beauty in everything – which I find very inspiring. She just made the most of every single day until she died.'

I took a deep breath. It was as though this bereaved and grieving daughter was articulating precisely what we hope to enable in a hospice – a state of living while dying in which, for all the larceny of serious illness, the beauty and comfort of the world still abound. I am not sure anything conveys the essence of palliative care quite like 'My Life's Stem Was Cut', one of Dunmore's final poems in which, though painfully aware of life's brevity, she describes her conscious decision to bloom while dying. The poem concludes with devastating simplicity:

I know I am dying
But why not keep flowering
As long as I can
From my cut stem?

Why indeed? It is a question none of us can answer with certainty until we face a terminal diagnosis ourselves. What I can say, though, from first-hand experience, is that for a place synonymous with dying, a hospice is remarkably full of life, in all its bittersweetness, simply going on.

10

Clutching at Straws

So let us not talk falsely now
The hour is getting late.

Bob Dylan, 'All Along the Watchtower'

When Finn, our son, was four years old, we – or rather, I – nearly lost him. It was a Saturday morning in winter, the least sensible time to brave the local supermarket, but we were out of milk and cornflakes, the empty fridge emblematic of two overwrought working parents, so Finn and I set off in the frost for emergency provisions.

Wrapped against the chill in hat, mittens, puffer jacket and wellies, he was desperate, as always, to talk about dinosaurs. Still at the age where his words could not always keep up with his thoughts, we discussed in fits and starts who would triumph in Spinosaurus versus Ankylosaurus and I made him giggle by inventing ever more outlandish uses for a Spinosaurus's spine. The morning was cold enough for him to blow smoke like a dragon, and his paw felt warm and soft in mine.

Inside the supermarket, I held that paw tight. Grim-faced families jostled their trolleys down the aisles, a kind of slow-motion demolition derby, with bumper packs of toilet roll and howling babies to dodge. Almost trotting with excitement, hand straining in mine, Finn tugged me towards his favourite aisle, the one stacked with the overpriced plastic tat that makes parents' hearts sink as their children plead for 'treats'. I steered him away through the sea of shoppers, their foreheads furrowed with the rhetorical question, did I really slog my guts out all week only to arrive at *this*?

I breathed a sigh of relief when we made it to the checkout. Trying to keep hold of Finn's hand in the crowd had been the parental equivalent of wrangling a lemur. As he gazed trans-fixed at the rows of child-baiting, cynically placed sweeties, a finger tracing their wrappers with reverence, I swiftly unloaded the contents of our basket. When I glanced back, he was gone.

'Finn?' I asked, looking back along the line of shoppers. 'Did any of you see which way he went, please?' I felt a prickle of irritation at the faces staring blankly back at me. But no anxiety, not yet. I knew where he would try to head.

Squeezing past the queuing trolleys, I looked left and right. No Finn, so I hurried to the children's gift aisle, the tuts of impatience from the till I had left possibly imagined, but more likely real. When I reached the toys and found the aisle empty, I felt the first tightness in my throat, the first lurch of sickness in my stomach. Where was he? How was he not here?

'Finn?' My voice sounded tight and thin. 'Finn?' I started striding back, retracing my steps, craning to glimpse his blue bobble hat between the teeming legs and trolleys. Accelerating now, breaking into a run, I bawled his name, fear flooding my larynx. 'Finn! Finn!' Louder, harsher. I could not think, I could not breathe. Fear was causing me to howl for my son – the sound of shameless desperation.

Somehow, in moments, the whole supermarket knew his name, that he was missing, and was four, and that his coat was bright blue. Fellow mothers looked strained, scanning the aisles. Then, a yell: 'Look! He's there!' Someone pointing towards the fish counter. 'There, there! With the security guard.' I half ran, half stumbled towards my son, who stood engrossed by a gleaming whole salmon lying wide-mouthed on the ice.

'Finn!' My voice, his name, was almost an accusation as I scooped him violently into my arms, crushing him tight to my chest. 'Thank you,' I cried to the guard, who was shifting awkwardly. Finn sobbed with fear as I buried my face in his hair. 'It's OK, it's OK. I'm sorry, darling. I was so worried. I thought I'd lost you.'

Slowly, we made our way back towards the checkouts. Someone had gathered our groceries back into their basket and dumped it on a stack of discounted washing powder. No longer the focus of drama and attention, we took our place at the back of the queue. Full of guilt first at losing him and then at yelling at him, I broke a supermarket rule and allowed Finn to choose some sweeties. He chewed contentedly as I endeavoured to ignore my racing heart and waited for the sickness to subside.

There is a violence to our longing not to lose those we love. When I tore through the supermarket, deranged with fear, my desperation, essentially, was a split-second, fifty-million-year descent to the deepest, oldest, most primal part of my brain controlling survival, instinct and drive. My limbic self, feathered and clawed, primed to fight with my last breath for my child. The animal within us all.

For all the seeming tranquillity of a hospice interior, the savagery of grief lurks just beneath the surface, and for this there is no palliation. Occasionally, it erupts in physical form. A brother, perhaps, pinning another against the wall, and then the call we hate to make, for the hospital security guards to come and contain the wildness unleashed. There may be wailing, shrieking, slamming of fists against concrete, someone hurling themselves to the floor, the total embodiment of heartbreak. Sometimes I have the same sensation at work as before the smash and roar of a stormy sea: if there is this much force in one wave, one person, then there is too much world for my brain to grasp, it is too stupefyingly powerful.

Perhaps surprisingly, the other kind of desperation – that of patients themselves not to relinquish their hold on life – less commonly seizes our ward. Usually, by the time someone reaches the hospice doors they have accepted, on some level, that they are going to die, however much this may frighten them. My colleagues – oncologists, haematologists, physicians, surgeons – will have typically already conducted those harrowing conversations in which a person's lingering hopes for cure are dispelled once and for all, often with great sensitivity. But not always. Even in a hospice, a place synonymous with dying, that role can fall to us.

When I met Joe for the first time, it was his apparent health, his veneer of vivacity, that took my breath away. Having read his notes, traced his scans on a screen, I knew that beneath the carapace of apparent flawlessness, his flesh was silently imploding. Joe was only thirty-six. A childhood in Kenya with expatriate parents had given him memories of wildebeest and lions, of teeming life on an endless savannah, of vast cathedrals of sky. But it had also sown the seeds of his premature destruction. African sunshine, gorgeous and deadly, had zeroed in on the cells of his skin, slashing and burning its DNA. Miniature breaks in his genetic code, first one mutation, and then another, had turned a single human cell into a deadly weapon, a proliferating force, ravenous and tenacious.

Joe noticed an odd blemish on his back that had begun to itch and ooze. Slowly, it staked a claim across his ribs like ink on blotting paper. Finally, Angie, his wife, insisted that her husband stop procrastinating and go to the doctor. Events unfurled with bewildering swiftness. Joe found himself facing the neon flare of theatre lights, the scalpel's sting, the biopsy confirming the surgeon's worst fears, and – what we strive to convince ourselves is only ever the fate of others – the dizzying descent into a hospital on red alert, acting fast, acting now, the NHS not wasting a second in its determined, heroic, hopeless efforts to save a healthy man in freefall.

Having long since returned to the dreary English skies under which he was born, Joe, now a father of two young girls, was diagnosed with malignant melanoma, the most aggressive and feared of skin cancers. Though the surgery to remove his tumour was swift and exhaustive, it was also, it turned out, to no avail. As so often with melanoma – the ultimate stealth operator – malignant cells still lurked in his blood, unseen, undetected, biding their time with reptilian patience. Just when Joe's three-year reprieve since his original diagnosis had lulled him into the tentative hope that maybe, just maybe, his melanoma was history, it declared its return with terrible abruptness. One moment he was sitting with his wife and girls eating spaghetti for dinner, the next he was keeling off his chair and slumping on the tiles, arms and legs jerking, eyes gyrating, drooling on to his T-shirt.

Joe's melanoma had spread from his skin to his brain. Though his seizures were swiftly controlled with anti-epileptic medications, neither drugs nor radiation nor even the latest gamma-knife surgery could obliterate the tumours that now clung there like crabs dug into rock. When I met him for the second time, on his arrival at the hospice, his health had been replaced by deathly exhaustion. Angie, a care worker, had been working flat out to pay the bills, while Joe struggled to look after their daughters. Though friends and family had rallied to support them, Joe's energy had waned so precipitously that the couple were now at breaking point.

'I don't want to be here. I need to get home as soon as possible,' Joe declared when I entered his room. 'I need to be building up my strength, get some weight back on, be strong enough for the girls and my immunotherapy.' Beside him, Angie sat with her eyes to the floor, tugging at threads on the sleeve of her jumper.

Joe's oncologists, I knew, had already concluded he could no longer withstand further treatment. His seizures had recurred, his tumours were spreading, his body was too frail to take any more. They had transferred him from their ward to the hospice to die, yet neglected to discuss this with their patient. I had been waiting all day for them to come and talk to him, the team he relied on and trusted.

'How soon before I'll get started?' asked Joe, almost childlike in his urgency. 'If it goes well with the immunotherapy, I'm going to get some more gamma knife too. But I have to start now. There's no time to waste.'

Angie, a slight young woman half the size of her husband, began to cry softly. I could see she did not believe a word of it. 'I've really got to get back to the girls,' she told me. 'I just can't wait here any more for Joe's oncologist.'

Two pairs of eyes were locked on mine, one full of hope, the other of tears. I longed with every fibre to be anywhere but here, pinned down by the weight of a life and its extinction. I could only imagine what filled Joe's mind in this moment. Perhaps his youngest's first day at school, his oldest's head teacher's award, the future mermaid birthday parties, the first battles over boyfriends, the summers spent in sand dunes, the snowball fights at winter – all of this life to come, to savour, moments dancing like charms on a string, yet unspooling without him, a father lost to cancer.

The temptation to leave this conversation to others almost overpowered me. I could frame any number of justifications in my head, pretending my abdication was in my patient's best interests. Instead, I steeled myself to prise a young father away from the life he still yearned for, the future he clung to so fiercely.

I took a deep breath and sat down. The external world fell away into shadow. Four eyes, out of time, were waiting and staring. We had arrived at the point where everything hangs in the balance.

The words you choose, in these moments, could not matter more. A misstep may spell irreparable damage. Gently, calmly, without pity or drama, I embarked on the task of cleaving my patient from his future, while striving to preserve something he could still believe in. It is a delicate dissection, the tallest of orders. But it can be done – because the life we have left is still life in all its loveliness, if only we can inhabit the present.

'Joe,' I began, 'the oncologists have seen how much weaker you've become in the last few weeks—'

'Yes,' he interrupted, 'but that's why I'm here. To build myself up again. To get strong enough for immunotherapy.' Even as he spoke, I could see how hard he was fighting to resist his exhaustion. I had to be blunt, choosing words without ambiguity.

'I'm sorry, Joe. That's not what they've told us. Immunotherapy can be really tough on the body, and we don't think you are strong enough to take any more of it.'

'You can fix that, though. You can get me stronger. That's what I'm here for. You can give me decent food, physiotherapy. I'll get better. Tell her, Angie. Tell her.'

I turned to Angie, whose head was in her hands, weeping quietly. I needed both of them to know she was in no way responsible for these decisions being made by her husband's doctors.

'Joe,' I continued, 'Angie wants you to live as much as you do. But there comes a point when we know you're too weak for more treatment. You're too exhausted. It wouldn't work for you.'

'You don't know that,' he insisted. 'You can't say that for certain. Let me try. Please don't take away my chances.'

I steeled myself to go on. 'Joe, if we tried more treatment now it would make you feel rotten. It might even shorten the time you have left. We can't cure your cancer or slow it down any more. But we can help you feel as well as you possibly can, to give you the best chance of enjoying every day as it comes with the girls and Angie.'

There was silence, the longest, darkest pause. All the advice for these conversations is that you must, without fail, use the word 'dying', but in Joe's case this felt like unnecessary bludgeoning. Like me, Angie waited quietly. The room felt very still. I wondered if Joe were starting to fall asleep in his bed, but behind closed eyes he was thinking, adapting, perhaps, even, accepting. Finally, as though dredging himself back from the underworld, he spoke in a voice little more than a whisper.

'Is there any chance at all of me getting out of here alive?'

I met his gaze without flinching. 'If you would like to spend your time at home then, yes, Joe, absolutely. We are here to try and help you live the time you have left on your terms, the way you want to. We can't stop your cancer, but we will do everything we can to support you, including going home, if you'd like to.'

I knew this was not what he meant. He wanted his whole future, a glimmer of life untruncated. But time was short, so few moments to cherish, and Joe was tortured by the desire to prolong them, chasing round after round of futile treatment. I did not want to crush all his hope. My job was to disillusion Joe sufficiently that he might find acceptance, while not completely devastating him.

'I'm dying,' he said at last.

'Yes, Joe,' I said softly, 'you are. But you still have time with Angie and the girls. That is precious, and we want to help you make the most of it. What really matters to you in the time you have left?'

Recalibrating your hopes – setting achievable goals such as reaching a child's birthday or a final Christmas – can bring great comfort. In Joe's case, his aims were simple: to spend as much time as he could with his wife and daughters. The conversation ended when his fatigue overwhelmed him. Angie and I retreated outside where, to my surprise, she thanked me. 'It had to be said,' she told me bluntly. 'He couldn't enjoy anything. He was so obsessed by treatment.' She paused for a moment. 'Would you talk to the girls tomorrow? They want to ask you some questions too.'

I quaked inside at the prospect. I wished I could say no, as if that were an option. The next morning, I sat inside a family room with Lottie, aged four, her big sister, Sarah, and their mother, who sat quietly as Sarah led the conversation.

'Why won't you give my dad more treatment?' she asked me with more gravity than a ten-year-old should ever need to muster. I soon discovered that this little girl with her hair still in bunches knew more about the management of intracranial metastatic melanoma than many doctors in my hospital. The questions kept coming like weapons.

'Immunotherapy isn't as tiring as chemotherapy, so why won't you let my dad have more of it?'

'Why won't gamma knife work this time if it worked last time for my dad?'

'If my dad wants to try something and he is going to die without it, then why aren't you just letting him try it?'

It was the hardest conversation I have ever experienced. The only thing that interrupted the barrage of questions were the sobs that burst from Sarah, sudden and explosive, after which she would wipe her cheeks dry, shake her head with impatience, and resume her interrogation. Each question was really the same question: *can't you give me something to hope for?* But her father was going to die and there was nothing anyone could do to prevent it. Patiently, gently, I dismantled every straw she clutched at until – as Peppa Pig honked and chortled from the smartphone clutched by Lottie – I found myself talking to this grief-stricken girl about cherishing the time she had left with her father. How she wished she could cuddle her daddy. How she would draw him pictures to brighten his room in the hospice. How much she wanted to make him smile. I had no idea if I was helping or hurting her. No one had taught me what to do here.

Our role, as palliative care doctors, is no longer the extension of life, the fight to stave off the inevitable. Acceptance of what cannot be controlled – working within, not against, the finality of terminal illness – enables us to focus on what we *can* influence. The quality, meaning and small joys of life, like the moments Joe enjoyed, cuddled up in bed with his daughters, in the days before he died.

These principles jar against the traditional medical model in which doctors do battle with death and disease, enabling humanity to triumph over what hurts or harms us. The history of medicine is, undeniably, a dizzying roll call of advances to celebrate. The first vaccines, antibiotics, chemotherapies, test tube babies, conscious neurosurgeries, titanium hips, bionic eyes, artificial hearts, transplanted faces. The list goes on and on. Even as I jot down these medical milestones, I cannot stop grinning with wonder and awe. The bloody-minded tenacity, the sheer ingenuity of those doctors and scientists – meaning that today we live longer and better than at any other point in human history.

But death cannot be defeated, and its deferment may come at a price. In striving to overcome illnesses, accidents, the brutal blows of chance, medicine has the power to extend our lives – but it can also, inadvertently, prolong human suffering. One person's desperately desired, life-extending treatment may be another's misery, a futile ordeal they come to wish their doctors had never inflicted. Time and again I encounter patients whose most heartfelt wish, at the end of their lives, is that they could swap the year of chemotherapies and surgeries they have just endured for a fraction of that time, lived free from gruelling side effects. 'You wouldn't flog a dead horse,' a patient once told me, 'except when the horse is human, and they happen to have cancer.'

In our era of cardiopulmonary resuscitation, artificial ventilation and long-term feeding through stomach tubes, life can endure and endure – but at what cost? Increasingly today, doctors question whether an over-interventionist approach to death – the medicalisation of mortality – is causing more harm than good. A defining question of modern medicine has therefore become not how do I keep this person alive, eking out more scraps of life, but *should* I?

Messy, complicated and ethically fraught dilemmas have replaced what used to be the simple inevitability of human dying. In an age of over-treatments that may burden a patient with side effects while failing to deliver the promised increments of extra life, how do we – doctors, patients, families, all of us − recognise the point at which it is time to stop striving and, instead, to let someone go? When, in short, is enough enough?

Once, when still a very junior doctor, I cared for a patient who, in his own words, for the last four months of his life had lived 'nothing but cancer, cancer, cancer'. Unlike the insidious trajectories of many early malignancies, in which a patient slowly declines with inexorable stealth, Henry Simpson was overwhelmed in the space of several hours. 'I woke up feeling normal,' he told me. 'But by the evening I knew something was seriously wrong. I actually thought I could be dying.'

From here, events unravelled with giddy alacrity. Rushed by ambulance to hospital in pain and delirium, his scans revealed a tumour encasing his ureters, the tubes connecting his kidneys to his bladder. Henry, at age fifty-two, had aggressive, invasive bowel cancer. Hastily − his failing kidneys were a life-threatening emergency − he was consented for the immediate insertion of stents, small plastic tubes that would allow his blocked kidneys once more to drain urine. Immediately after the procedure, Henry's oncologists now proposed radical surgery to remove the cancerous bowel and its surroundings. 'I felt like I had no choice,' he remembered. 'I signed the consent form, but really, if I'd known what would happen from then onwards, I never would have agreed to surgery.'

Though Henry survived the operation, he was left with a stoma. His faeces now drained into a bag attached to the outside of his belly. Over several weeks in hospital he gradually replaced the weight he had lost, beginning to approach the fitness required to start chemotherapy. But then, abruptly, his kidneys failed a second time. Cancer had again blocked his renal tract. Now, yet more tubes were inserted. One attached to each kidney, each draining urine out of his side into another plastic bag – a total of three surgical orifices.

By the time I met him, Henry was criss-crossed with scars, prone to endless infections, and thoroughly sick of it all. Still, I did not foresee what came next. 'Take them out,' he instructed. 'I never knew what I was signing up to. Just take the damn things out.'

I struggled to hold his gaze. 'If we take out the tubes, your kidneys will fail,' I said carefully, hunting deliberately for words devoid of ambiguity. 'You would die soon afterwards. It may be impossible to reverse that. I need to make sure you understand that this decision may cause you to die very quickly.'

'Look,' replied Henry, exasperated, 'I was dying the moment I was first diagnosed. It's just that no one ever gave me the chance to think about it. This is exactly what I never wanted to happen to me. Four months of hell in hospital.'

While the risks and benefits of his various operations had ostensibly been explained to him, at no point had Henry really taken any of it in. Nor had a doctor ever asked him the really critical questions. How much are you willing to endure for a chance of staying alive? What kind of being alive do you think you can tolerate? How much can you bear to be diminished? He had felt steamrollered by his doctors into a pointless ordeal – months of painful and degrading procedures at the behest of others who believed they knew what was best for him.

During lengthy conversations with various members of his medical team, spread out over a number of days, Henry's resolve was unwavering. He clearly had the capacity to make this decision for himself. The tubes in his kidneys, he insisted over and over, simply had to come out. It fell to me, his ward doctor, to remove them.

That morning, I arrived at work full of trepidation. But Henry was resolute. 'Right then, let's get on with it.' With a little tugging, a twist, and a snip of a surgical stitch, the first tube came away in my hands. A minute later, and another tube was out.

Although we had respected his wishes – allowed him to exercise control over the course of his cancer for perhaps the only time since its diagnosis – I brooded, feeling troubled and uncertain about what I had done. Deeply ingrained in my medical psyche was the urge to treat, to cure, to fix, to save. Resisting that impulse felt like a violation of my training as a doctor. Slowly, inexorably, once the tubes were out, Henry deteriorated, becoming increasingly delirious as toxins from his kidneys polluted his bloodstream. A week or so later, he died, precisely as he had intended. I was not prepared for how wrong doing the right thing could feel.

For all the triumphs and heroics of modern-day medicine, Henry's story illustrates its potential for dragging out and debasing the experience of dying. There is even a new name for this relentless over-treatment: 'desperation oncology'. It refers to the temptation to try even those treatments whose chances of success are vanishingly small, regardless of their side effects.

If, in striving for longer and better living, doctors end up merely prolonging your painful demise, then medicine has surely lost its way. But what if Henry had lived? With hindsight, the futility of his ordeal is obvious. Yet at the time, the hope, the prize, was eradication of the cancer that would otherwise kill him. At only fifty-two, he had stood to be cheated out of so much unlived future. Is clutching at straws so very unreasonable when you burn with every fibre to live?

These days, a powerful argument, made increasingly frequently, is that the greatest barrier to getting this balance right – and hence of dying 'well', or as closely as possible to the manner of our choosing – is silence. Our reluctance to talk openly and honestly about the risks and benefits of life-prolonging treatments, the potential costs of each attempt at cure, leaves patients in the dark, prone to blundering unawares into a relentlessly medicalised last experience of living.

In Britain, 82 per cent of the population have strong views about how they would like to be treated at the end of their lives, yet only 4 per cent of us have set out our wishes in a legally binding way, by writing an 'advanced directive'. Preparing for our own deaths in advance may be daunting, disturbing and – for some of us, doctors included – unthinkable. But it is, at least, a means of ensuring our wishes are known and respected at a time when we may no longer be able to communicate them. Deferring these discussions may mean that, when our time comes, we have missed our chance to shape and influence the manner of our dying. We might, for example, end our days on a ventilator, in an ITU-induced coma, when what we had always hoped for, yet never voiced, was to die at home, surrounded by our loved ones. How can patients hope to author the way their stories end if the conversation about all the possibilities never happens?

An analogy is sometimes drawn between modern and Victorian attitudes to sex and dying. The Victorians, the argument goes, were superb at discussing death but, for them, sex was strictly taboo, whereas we never stop pouring forth about sex yet dare not speak death's name. We feel the need to talk euphemistically – about 'passing on' or 'losing' someone – about the only event in our lives we can guarantee, with absolute certainty, is going to happen to every single one of us. Arguably, the messy matter of contemporary human dying requires us all, but especially doctors, to face up to our fears, look death in the eye and start admitting once more that we are mortal.

Everywhere these days – in newspaper columns, television documentaries and social media campaigns – people are being urged to talk about dying. In the UK and the US, for example, 'Death Cafés' have proliferated in which participants come together to 'drink tea, eat cake and discuss death'. More provocatively, 'Beyond' – a price comparison website for funeral parlours – caused outrage in Britain in 2018 when it sought to increase its online traffic through a particularly brash series of billboard advertisements. In one, a sun-kissed young couple frolicked through waves on a sandy beach, clutching not surfboards but two-dimensional wooden coffins. The advert, designed to mimic a pitch for a cheap package holiday, screamed shrill slogans for no-frills cremation: 'All-inclusive . . . roasting temperatures . . . depart from anywhere . . . once in a lifetime'. The company maintained it had designed deliberately irreverent advertisements to start a national conversation about death and burial costs, with co-founder Ian Strang boldly asserting in an interview: 'We're stripping away the emperor's clothes, the over-reverence assigned to what is, after all, an inevitable conclusion, an inescapable purchase – using humour. We're turning up the volume to ten in the hope it paves the way for everyone else to at least make it to five – planting a flag and saying, "Here's permission to talk about death."'

The word 'purchase' here is telling. When I read Strang's words, still raw and dazed after my own father's death, I longed to respond in Anglo-Saxon expletives. It is one thing to advocate sincerely the value of confronting our taboos around death, but quite another to use brash, crass, clickbait ads to monetise people's fears of dying. The last thing, surely, bereaved people need is companies co-opting a narrative of frankness in order to turn a quick profit?

Opening up about dying can, of course, be immensely valuable. Many hospice patients, for example, are overwhelmed with relief when given space to talk fully and frankly about their own imminent deaths, after endless conversations with family members full of veils and euphemisms. But doctors learn early on in their careers that merely urging their patients to change their behaviours is a strategy doomed to failure. The more stridently we demand compliance with our wishes, the greater the likely resistance. After all, there is nothing more annoying than being told what's good for you, especially by a know-all who uses words like pseudohypoparathyroidism.

Personally, things I don't like to talk or think about include:

Global warming
This year's tax return
The state of the attic
The rise of far right populism
The number of emails in my inbox
My future being beset by (at best) decrepitude and frailty

The day when my children stop climbing into bed
   for cuddles
The menopause
Pensions
Declining numbers of hedgehogs and bees

I am not 'in denial' about these topics, but nor do I choose to ruminate on any of them. This January, I will doubtless scramble, as every year, to complete a tax return in time, and one day – perhaps next year – I will clear the attic. Similarly, it is entirely possible to be fully aware of one's own mortality while preferring not to engage in thoughts of dying. This does not automatically elevate death to taboo status. Maybe, more prosaically, dying is on a par with tax returns and pensions. We know we should address them all proactively, it is just that the admin involved is, frankly, tiresome.

At the risk of undermining my own credibility, I feel duty-bound to confess a failing. For all my experience of palliative medicine, for all my knowledge of the suffering that can occur when someone is horribly injured without an advance directive in place, setting out one's wishes in the event of serious illness, I have not quite managed to write my own directive. Nor, at any point, did my father. He loathed admin too. This means, were I one day to suffer catastrophic brain damage, ending up being kept alive by a mechanical ventilator, for example, there is no legal document detailing my passionate wish for no life-prolonging heroics. My husband and sister are fully aware I would want the plug pulled, preferring swift oblivion to a tubed, gowned, twilight existence. But nowhere have I written this down – and indolence, not fear, is the culprit. (By the time this book is published I *will* have got around to it, but not for one second will I ever disapprove of someone who has not.)

Even when denial does define our relationship with dying, this is not necessarily a bad thing. Indeed, it may be an essential component of how a patient copes, psychologically, with their fate. Once, in the hospice, I cared for a magnificently forthright 102-year-old whose ferocious intelligence kept us all on our toes. A former economist for whom numbers were a lifelong passion, Professor Bonicci's own mortal arithmetic was strictly out of bounds. She arrived so diminished and gaunt from heart failure I could have scooped her up in my arms and carried her to her bed myself. Each gentle invitation to explore her prognosis was firmly and impatiently rebuffed. She preferred to discuss John Maynard Keynes and Milton Friedman. My morning ward round began to resemble an Oxbridge tutorial until, one day, as I was leaving, she suddenly said, 'One more thing, Dr Clarke.'

I paused, returned to her bedside, and waited.

'I'd like to ask you a question,' she began.

This is it, I thought triumphantly. At last we were going to have that conversation.

'Do you think . . . ' she continued awkwardly. 'Do you think it is possible that . . . well . . . '

I waited.

'That I may not have an enormously long time to live?'

Professor Bonicci, part of me longed to exclaim, *you are 102 years old. Of course you don't have long to live! You are in your second century of life!* But all she would allow me to do was murmur the briefest assent.

'Thank you, that is all,' she replied, cutting me off before I could utter the D-word. 'You may go now.'

Dismissed from her bedside, I could not help but smile. The next day, we were back to macroeconomics. When she died, a few days later, at peace in her sleep, I wondered whether extreme denial could itself be life-prolonging. Perhaps her resolute refusal to acknowledge her finitude was the very thing that had propelled Professor Bonicci into longevity.

Rather than telling people they *must* talk about dying, and insisting that they use non-euphemistic language to do so – 'death', 'dying', 'reclaiming the D-word' – I prefer to take as my starting point the principle that, in matters as personal as confronting our mortality, each of us should do it our way. There is no one 'right' way to converse about death; instead, this is a matter of individual preference. Doctors can and should set a straight-talking example, but, if our aim is for everyone to end their lives humanely, then words are only part of the problem. Addressing, for example, the hard matter of resources – sufficient doctors, nurses, carers and therapists to ensure patients with terminal illness have the choice to live at home, hospice or hospital with equal comfort and dignity – is at least as vital.

A few months after specialising in palliative medicine, I began to believe I had this death thing licked. It was not that it was easy – far from it – but that, whatever a day at work threw at me, I was reasonably confident of knowing how to help, or of knowing someone else in the team who could. The hospice was not some blackened wasteland, torched by wildfires of grief.

'Do you find it depressing?' Dad asked me one day, always keen to ensure his children were happy.

'No, Dad, not at all. I love it. I can't wait to get started in the morning.'

The passion in my answer surprised me, but not my father. What had sapped his joie de vivre, towards the end of his career, was not his immersion in other people's distress but being slowly ground down by an unmanageable workload. What had reinvigorated him, time and again, were the moments of connection with his patients, the experience of sharing the pains, fears, hopes and dreams that, knitted together, make us human. Now I was fortunate enough, every day at work, to have the same privilege.

As for my former concerns that being surrounded by death might somehow, cumulatively, leach the life from me, the opposite was true. Nothing throws longevity into sharper relief than other people's lives cut short. As a woman with the luxury of four whole decades of life behind her, I knew precisely how lucky I was. The slow sag of flesh, the start of wrinkled decrepitude, these were things to embrace with lusty gratitude. If a friend lamented their lost bloom of youth, well, I would try to be diplomatic and hide my frustration, but I knew that grey hairs and reading specs were gifts, not curses, and wasting time on appearance a folly. Ageing was neither a right nor a challenge, nor something to fend off: it was a privilege.

In the year of my birth, 1972, the American writer Henry Miller marked his entry into the ninth decade of life by publishing an extraordinary essay on the subject of ageing. I particularly enjoy his dim view, in *On Turning Eighty*, of the hubris of medical science:

With all the progress medicine has made over the years we still have a pantheon of incurable diseases. The germs and microbes seem to have the last word always. When all else fails the surgeon steps in, cuts us to pieces, and clears us out of our last penny. And that's progress for you.

Today, as doctors, ethicists, journalists and the public debate the unintentional harms of desperation medicine, Miller's stance looks remarkably prescient. But what moves me the most in the essay are his reflections on the most incurable disease of them all, the state of being mortal. The true metric of youthfulness, Miller argues, is a matter not of time but of attitude:

If at eighty you're not a cripple or an invalid, if you have your health, if you still enjoy a good walk, a good meal (with all the trimmings), if you can sleep without first taking a pill, if birds and flowers, mountains and sea still inspire you, you are a most fortunate individual and you should get down on your knees morning and night and thank the good Lord for his savin' and keepin' power. If you are young in years but already weary in spirit, already on the way to becoming an automaton, it may do you good to say to your boss – under your breath, of course – 'Fuck you, Jack! You don't own me!' … If you can fall in love again and again, if you can forgive your parents for the crime of bringing you into the world, if you are content to get nowhere, just take each day as it comes, if you can forgive as well as forget, if you can keep from growing sour, surly, bitter and cynical, man you've got it half licked.

For me, there is nothing in this world more life-affirming than working with patients close to life's end whose sense of wonder, like Miller's, remains intact. I am surrounded at work by patients who have never loved life more fiercely and who, by rights, you could argue, should be consumed by bitterness. But, so often the opposite is true. Life, somehow, wins out. Shortly before he died, one patient, Peter, captured the anguish and ache of it perfectly: 'I love my wife. I love my daughter. I love every single thing about this world.' The yearning in those words was almost unbearable to hear and yet, as he said them, he was smiling. Later, too weak to leave his hospice bed, Peter – a dying man who knew it – would raise his eyes to the trees outside and paint watercolours of the birds at his window. His pictures, propped on his bedside table, brought the life he ached not to lose inside the room he would never leave. He ended his days still living, still loving, still creating. And I am not sure you get more inspirational than that.

Deeply immersed now in the life of the hospice, I loved the team I had become a part of and the ethos, shared by us all, that dying is a part of living, and that the terminally ill are no less deserving of care and attention than anyone else in a hospital. Then, a few months into my palliative medicine, the phone rang. It was Dad.

'Are you free to speak, Rachel?' he asked. I lied. I was certain, the moment I heard the strain in his voice, that he was about to say something terrible. I was on the school run, jammed in rush-hour traffic, suddenly wired with foreboding. His voice filled the car, thin and crackly on speakerphone. 'I'm afraid I have some bad news.'

I knew. I felt it take my breath away. He did not need to say the word 'cancer'. For months now he had mentioned the odd twinge of pain, a mild griping and grumbling in his belly.

Always downplayed, always carefully framed in the innocuous context of a predisposition to abdominal cramping, the result of a benign and common condition, diverticulitis. I saw in a flash what he had been seeking to elicit – the reassurance from his doctor-daughter that would salve his own physician's unease, that the niggle was something more sinister lurking, that special, telling, doctor's doubt we both knew so well, and both had used, on occasion, to save our patients' lives. Now Dad was the patient and I had failed him. How eagerly I had taken his cues at face value, as hungry as him to discount the ominous. The lack of red flags, the absence of grave features that he knew, precisely, how to signal to me. A *folie à deux*, doctor to doctor, both of us constructing the narrative we wanted and had chosen to assume was true. *Oh my God*, I silently screamed. *In what have we both been complicit?*

Gripping the wheel, I fought the prickles of fear at the base of my neck and struggled to convey a tone of lightness. 'Go on, Dad. What's happened?'

'I've been diagnosed with bowel cancer.' A pause. His own monumental effort at calmness. 'Quite a large tumour, by the look of it today in endoscopy. I'll be having a staging CT next week.'

We both knew better than to serve up platitudes. There was nothing reassuring a scan could offer, merely the absence of worse news. Major surgery loomed, chemotherapy, indignity. The parameters of awfulness were yet to be defined but sat in a dish containing water and formaldehyde, soon to be mounted in wax for posterity, the cancer – the fucker – its cells and deformities to be slavishly scrutinised by doctors other than me, the beady-eyed ones with the microscopes. Everything now hinged on those slivers of flesh and their degree of freakishness. Even cancers that have colonised distant parts of the body – Stage 4, the diagnosis doctors hate to give, for there is no Stage 5, only death – can sometimes be curable. But the grade, the deviancy of the cancerous cells in a biopsy, correlates with the speed and aggression of their assault upon a body. I was all too aware of the irony here. Those cells would now be preserved in a pathologist's vault for a decade, their longevity guaranteed, while Dad's prognosis, his lifespan, hung in the balance.

'Dad, you are not your average seventy-four-year-old. You can walk twenty miles. You climb mountains. You know this matters, you're strong,' I told him. And it did. But it was also barely relevant.

'I know, I know, Rachel. But, of course, it's the grade that's the thing. And whether the scan shows metastases,' he replied.

I had pulled into the car park of my daughter's school and was crouching over the wheel. 'I'm so sorry, Dad, I have to go or I'm going to be late for Abbey.' We said our goodbyes. There was only one thing left. 'Dad, I love you.'

His voice cracked a little as he replied. 'I love you too, dear. Try not to worry too much.'

Life, of course, never pauses. I hurled the phone into the footwell of the car, wiped my face with the back of my hand, and stepped out into the cacophony of several hundred children, high as kites with liberation, hurtling and screaming across the playground.

'Rach, are you OK?' someone asked me. My friend, another mother, brow furrowed with concern.

'No,' I muttered, face crumpling. 'Dad has cancer.'

Other mothers scooped up Abbey with their own, distracting

her with raisins and chocolate while I wrestled, round the corner, to compose myself. It was the start of a future avalanche of kindnesses. People, I would think that night, wrung out from all the crying, can be so exceptionally lovely. For now, gritted teeth and dry eyes were required. I heard a shriek and tiny footsteps thumping. There she was, my daughter, my diminutive stampeder, leaping into my arms like a feral force of nature, scattering words in every direction. What life, I thought, as I tickled and kissed her, my tears staining her school jumper. What astonishing, miraculous vivacity.

11

The Price of Love

No one ever told me that grief felt so like fear.

C. S. Lewis, *A Grief Observed*

Everything has changed. The hospice, a place I entered so eagerly, proud to be part of its collective endeavour to offer solace and comfort at the end of life, has mutated from sanctuary into minefield. Without constant vigilance, every step guarded, I know I can be ambushed from any direction.

The scan, inevitably, showed spread. In keeping with its grade – the worst, it turns out, the most hungry and virulent – my father's cancer has already laid claim to his liver. He will have surgery, then chemotherapy, to buy him some time, but the conclusion is almost certainly set in stone.

My patients are now the face of Dad's future. This jaundice, this pain, these thinly papered ribs and sternum, all of it is coming for him, I know it. There are particular patients I dread. These are the ones in the hinterland between life and death, unconscious yet warm, silent yet breathing, still here, still quivering with the last beats of life, yet already lost to their loved ones. I cannot bear to imagine my father cut adrift in this space, lost between life and its extinction, both here and forever departed.

Briefly, superstition trumps science. Late at night, I start to imagine that in thinking these thoughts, I might somehow enact them, consigning my father to the fate of my patients. The personal and professional in queasy collusion, each bleeding into the other. 'Get a grip,' I tell myself. 'Your patients deserve better than this.'

In lieu of sleep, I attempt nocturnal logic. *Look, there is no breaking news here, nothing remotely tragic. A seventy-four-year-old man has been diagnosed with cancer. With one in two of us facing precisely that fate, it really doesn't get more banal.*

I know that Dad's life is largely behind him, decades of rich, lived experience. Calamity is not this, it is a child erased before they even unfurled, or a baby who dies in neonatal intensive care before they ever learn to speak or walk or see the world outside the hospital. New life is supposed to hold boundless potential: here is where tragedy lies. Except that, on this occasion, the patient is my father. And, as I am swiftly discovering, grief, like love, resists reason. The mortal calculus of who deserves pity is fraudulent. Love makes a mockery of bean counting.

Shamefaced, I think back on prior judgements I have airily made – my hierarchy, if you will, of what counts as true tragedy. Young children, clearly, outranked everyone. How could anything compare to the heart-wrecking horror of losing a child? Then, on becoming a doctor, I soon discovered the pain of loss at life's other extreme. Those timeless couples, wedded for sixty-odd years, who can scarcely remember life without the other, and who would rather die than outlive them. Surely only the most callous mathematics could compute their grief as undeserving?

Nevertheless, the judgements persisted. When I turned forty, I liked to joke with friends that this was it, I had officially outlived the period during which I was young enough to earn a doctor's sympathy. 'No, seriously,' I would say, laughing but insistent. 'Once you're out of your thirties, you don't deserve any pity. You're lucky – you've lived a decent lifetime.'

One day in the hospice, a fraught Friday evening, I had found myself seething with anger. In one room, a young woman lay dying. Her husband and her parents sat beside her, quietly united in loss. Her children were tucked up at home with their auntie, two toddlers carefully sequestered away from the fog of grief surrounding their mother. Next door was another patient, a woman in her late nineties. Crammed into this room were, I suppose, fifteen or twenty family members. A raucous bunch, devoted to their matriarch, their vigil was loud and rowdy. Earlier in the day I had hovered outside the door, on the brink of entering to plead for sensitivity towards the other hospice patients and families.

Suddenly, a collective howl filled the corridor. An ear-splitting bellow that grew only louder as hysterical mourners spilled from the room, shrieking and collapsing in heaps on linoleum. The sound was as ugly as it was deafening. I hardly dared imagine what the young woman's family was thinking, so close to this apocalyptic wailing. The urge to protect my patients made me fierce. *Yes, OK, she's died!* I wanted to yell back at the wailers. *Two years off a hundred. What a rare and magnificent innings. Now, for the love of God, will you please stop terrifying the still living? Show some thought for others.*

How easy it is to judge what you have never experienced. My kneejerk hostility was born out of ignorance. Now here I am, a few weeks down the line, having turned overnight from someone who assumed – naively – she knew better than most how to face death unflinchingly into a frantic, desperate, flailing mess. *Rach, you're a palliative care doctor, for heaven's sake.* Yet for all my professional exposure to grief, of helping other people navigate matters of living and dying, nothing has prepared me for the shock of recognition that cancer will kill my father.

Objectively doctoring by day – or trying to – I fret the nights away clutching at straws. 'A trial,' I mutter, obsessively scouring the internet for snake oil. Gone are the doctor's scientific appraisal skills, supplanted by wishful thinking. *All those amazing new immunotherapies. The monoclonals. The new CTLA-4 inhibitors. There must be a trial drug out there that can transform this, give him his life back, give me back my dad.* The ferocity of this longing not to lose him obliterates, at times, both my training and my reason. I just do not want him to die.

I talk to my colleagues, explain the situation. After a few days, I reach an uneasy equilibrium. You must get on with doing what you can for your patients, I tell myself. You cannot save them either, but you can still help, and you have to keep trying. One thing is certain. All those years of medical training, I now know, have singularly failed to equip me with proper insight into the magnitude of other people's grief, and of our desperation to keep our loved ones with us, here, now, just a little longer.

*

The sky has the brittle gleam of ice about it. Up there, in the thinnest film of blue, a red kite is lazily slicing through ozone. As we step out of the car, the crunch of boots on frost and gravel, its casual aerobatics catch Dad's eye.

'Dave would approve,' he tells me, turning his head on one side to savour the deftly tilting wings and tail of a virtuoso aviator.

'He certainly would,' I smile.

We stand still for a moment, eyes glued to the sky, admiring the kite's precision manoeuvres.

'Christ, it's cold,' says my brother, bringing us back down to earth.

'Come on then,' says Dad. 'If anyone should be moaning about the cold, I should.' The chemotherapy has attacked the nerves in his extremities, making him exquisitely sensitive to cold, which now he feels as lancing pains in his fingertips.

'Well, get your woolly hat on then, mister,' I chide him.

Grumbling, my father sets off across the car park towards what is, quite frankly, an architectural monstrosity, a mash-up of the baroque with Victorian Gothic and a splash of mock Tudor for good measure. 'Jesus,' he declares, 'what a fucking carbuncle.'

I grin happily. Dad's finest hour, when it comes to swearing, was when Finn, then four years old, returned from a weekend away at my parents and, upon inhaling one whiff of the noxious nappy his baby sister had just filled, exclaimed, 'Jesus wept, Abbey! What in the name of Christ are you doing?' Forty-eight hours in the company of his granddad, and already a seasoned blasphemer.

Dad, my brother and I have come to Bletchley Park in

Buckinghamshire, the mansion famously commandeered during the Second World War to house nearly ten thousand government codebreakers. Our day trip, inspired by his cancer, is taking me back to my childhood. The intelligence services set about staffing the park's sprawling grounds and prefabricated wooden huts with pretty much anyone with a brain they could lay their hands on: cryptographers, linguists, mathematicians, astronomers – even, when push came to shove, women.

Bletchley had a reputation for ramshackle chaos. Homemade codebreaking machines were literally held together with sticking tape and pieces of string. One was even named 'Heath Robinson'. Somehow, this ragbag of brilliant eccentrics, led by Alan Turing, ended up cracking Enigma, the most notorious of all the German military ciphers, and shortening the war by an estimated two years. Dad, a lifelong lover of military history, has always wanted to visit. Halfway through six cycles of chemotherapy, there is absolutely no time like the present.

We traipse happily from one freezing single-storey wooden hut to another, our breath condensing in the air around us. Dad devours it all with characteristic enthusiasm. Nothing about him is cancerous. We love the Bakelite telephones, the uniforms, enamel mugs and clunky proto-computers. Most of all, we are seduced by the peculiarly British romance of a crack team of maverick geniuses, muddling through in what are, essentially, oversized garden sheds, yet somehow still saving the day.

The German Enigma cipher, we learn, was a fiendishly ingenious system of codes based on five-figure groups. It was deemed by the Germans, from mathematical first principles no less, to be impossible to break – provided it was used properly. The fatal flaw, revealed at Bletchley, lay not in the code but in its operators. Human beings being human, matters of the heart crept in. Some of the German cipher clerks broke the rules by using their wives' or girlfriends' names in their call signs, or by repeating certain phrases at the beginning and end of their messages. Each was a chink of light to the codebreakers through which, slowly but surely, the entire, elaborate edifice of Enigma began to unravel.

For a moment, I think of the code hardwired inside the cells of my father's body. A, C, G, T. Adenine, cytosine, guanine, thymine – four simple nucleotides, the bedrock of our DNA, that have dictated every nuance of his lifetime. Infinitely more impressive than even the boffins of Bletchley is the extraordinary fact that, for over seventy years, the thirty-seven trillion cells of his body have teemed and divided, all the while replicating their inner code perfectly, every error and glitch corrected or destroyed.

Then, one day, invisible and silent, came the one in thirty-seven trillion mutation. A single cell, deep inside my father's guts, whose mismatched code refused to die, and who, in genetic defiance of his body's checks and balances, began to spawn more of its own. One cell with immortal ambition. On and on its sons and daughters go – a ruthless, unstoppable, territorial grab that is underway even now, as Dad walks and talks beside me, a blitzkrieg by cells that will keep on living until they cause their host to die.

I stand for a while in front of Stephen Kettle's life-size sculpture of Alan Turing. The father of modern computing and artificial intelligence, the man who may have turned the course of a world war, sits pensively before one of his codebreaking machines. He was killed, of course, by an altogether different malignancy, the homophobia of his time. When Turing confessed his 'gross indecency' – homosexuality – to the police, he was spared prison only after agreeing to chemical castration. With his security clearance revoked and all intelligence work over, he was found dead of cyanide poisoning in his home two years later, a half-eaten apple beside him.

The statue is crafted from half a million pieces of Welsh slate, each of them five hundred million years old. As black and austere as space or mathematics, it speaks of impenetrability: I am looking into black holes, deep time, things I cannot grasp. Against these scales of millions and trillions – the dimensions of cells, codes, oncology, geology – one human life feels as insubstantial as air. The numbers swim, I bite my lip, tears are pricking at the corners of my eyes.

'Where have you been?' Dad suddenly asks, materialising at my shoulder. 'Come on, we haven't been to Hut 16 yet.'

My brother, I note, is trailing listlessly behind him, like a small boy on a school trip through the local cement factory. I start to laugh as we follow Dad's lead, trotting off through the frost towards another wooden hut that will not, I am fairly confident, be discernibly different to the last. All our family holidays were an exercise in dragging. Dad would haul us through bogs, up mountains, into blizzards, down scree. Dissent was futile, whinging even more so, tears whipped away by the wind. Only when strictly, absolutely necessary was a square of Kendal mint cake produced for frank refusals – *I am not going to walk another step! I don't care what you say! I hate you!* – to bribe his flouncing, feeble offspring in their sodden school cagoules up to the summit and back down again.

'Hey, does this remind you of the Lake District?' I murmur to my brother.

'It is exactly like the Lake District,' he laments. 'We've been looking inside huts for three hours straight. How does he have the energy? Is this normal?'

'Well,' I begin, considering my patients, 'not really normal for metastatic cancer and chemotherapy, no, but for him, I'd say, business as usual.'

Eventually, Dad has exhausted what Bletchley Park has to offer. In no sense is this relationship reciprocated. We sit in Hut 4, the former naval intelligence codebreaking hut that now, mercifully, houses the café, and chat over sandwiches about Alan Turing. It has been a beautiful day. Dad's face is aglow as he laughs with his children. You would never know that beneath the sleeve of that grubby fleece is a peripherally inserted central catheter, snug, veiled and quietly poised to mainline more of the cytotoxic poisons straight to the margin of his heart.

Back at work, I saw everything afresh. In particular, the way the weight of uncertainty bore down upon my patients' families. Two questions seemed to burden almost every loved one. How long? And, what will it be like when it happens? I had always sought to answer these as fully as I could, but now this felt like a professional imperative. The easy default – a cursory, mumbled, apologetic 'don't know' – had long seemed to me to be a doctorly cop-out. Usually, we did know, or at least we suspected. Never infallible, always liable to misjudgement, we could at least offer estimates of prognosis based on years of experience that patients and families lacked. For loved ones trapped in limbo, something was better than nothing, I believed, provided it was suitably caveated.

As for what actually happens when we die, historically, this moment of transition has vexed generations of doctors. In 1907, for example, a physician from Massachusetts, Dr Duncan MacDougall, sought to demonstrate the first scientific proof of the existence of the human soul by recording a loss of body weight – assumed to represent the departure of the soul – after death. MacDougall hypothesised that souls have physical weight and attempted to measure the change in mass of six patients at the moment of dying. One of the six patients lost three-quarters of an ounce, or 21.3 grams, leading to the research being popularised as the '21 grams experiment'.

Needless to say, MacDougall's methods raised eyebrows. Quite apart from the ethics of rigging dying patients' beds up on scales, a scientific sample size of one really does not cut it. Nor should the five patients without a deathbed weight loss have been conveniently discounted. And then there was the awkward matter of the dogs. The control arm of MacDougall's experiment appears to have been canine in nature – fifteen healthy dogs, poisoned in the name of science, none of which lost any weight after death, presumably on account of their soullessness. These limitations notwithstanding, the *New York Times* broke the story in an article entitled 'Soul Has Weight, Physician Thinks', and from that moment on the idea of a soul weighing 21 grams was forever cemented in popular culture.

Evidence of the enduring appeal of the soul's flight at the point of death is tucked away inside the Henry Ford museum in Michigan. There lies a test tube, sealed with paraffin, said to contain the last breath – the escaping soul – of Thomas Edison, the American inventor of the light bulb. Henry Ford was an employee of Edison's Illuminating Company, working his way up to become its chief engineer. An avid inventor himself, Ford worked in his spare time on designs that would eventually translate into the Model T Ford, the world's first affordable automobile. The two became devoted friends. Legend has it that when, in 1931, Edison became terminally ill, Ford asked Edison's son, Charles, to sit by the dying inventor's bedside holding a test tube next to his father's mouth to catch his final breath.

Charles later wrote of his father: 'Though he is mainly remembered for his work in electrical fields, his real love was chemistry. It is not strange, but symbolic, that those test tubes were close to him at the end. Immediately after his passing I asked Dr Hubert S. Howe, his attending physician, to seal them with paraffin. He did. Later I gave one of them to Mr. Ford.'

The test tube was lost for many years but then, in 1978, it resurfaced inside a cardboard tube labelled 'Edison's Last Breath?' Since then, the test tube has been on display in the museum, a testament to the enduring power of friendship, if not necessarily a soul captured within glass for eternity.

From the lofty perspective of modern medicine, the notion of death occurring at the point of the soul's departure might seem quaint and ridiculous. We doctors do not deal in such ethereal fancies. We insist on definitions that are rooted in evidence, in hard flesh and blood, and death is delineated by absences, not an invented presence. Over the years I have verified many scores of deaths, carefully documenting in patients' notes what is no longer there, the bleak poetry of human expiration:

No audible breath or heart sounds for greater than
  three minutes.
No palpable pulse for greater than three minutes.
Pupils are fixed, dilated and unreactive to light.
There is no palpable pacemaker.
There is no response to painful stimulus.
The patient has died.

Always – my nod to the enormity of a person's passing, my
reminder to myself that I am human and not merely doctor – I
carefully add the patient's name and a sentiment: 'May she rest
in peace.' I mean it. You need something to haul yourself back
from the supreme act of deviancy of hovering for an age over a
gaping-mouthed corpse, stethoscope listening to the sound of
silence, hand feeling for a pulse that has been forever stilled. A
disturbingly intimate yet lonely experience – just you and the
dead, privately communing behind polyester curtains. Three
minutes rarely feel longer.

But, just as the 21 gram hypothesis has been superseded, so
too has medical death – an apparent absolute – been reshaped
and redefined with time. No longer, in the twenty-first century, are the rhythms of blood and breath the essence of life.
Now, it is cerebral electricity, our brainwaves, that matter.
You can be pulseless, breathless, cyanotic, still, and yet, if the
right currents ebb and flow through grey matter, you live, you
inhabit this world. Clever machines can perform all the brute
functions of living – circulating your blood, inflating your
lungs, slowly funnelling liquid food through a tube in your
neck. Life support is a matter of basic mechanics, much of it
hinging on plumbing.

The terrible converse is also true. We can be dead while appearing entirely unblemished. Which is how, in a hospital ITU, a pair of stunned and bewildered parents may find themselves staring at their teenaged son – just hours after the bike ride he undertook without his helmet, unable to resist the tug of wind through his hair – and every single thing they see contravenes the fact that they have lost him. He is warm, flushed, intact, athletic. His cheeks are pink, there is no blood anywhere. The rise and fall of the dome of his chest, it has the beauty and lustre of youth about it. How can anyone dare to suggest this is not sleeping? Surely, in a moment, his eyes must open?

If brain death – a state arising from a brain injury so catastrophic that even the most vegetative of a body's functions must be delivered through the suck and hiss of machines – has existed only since the 1970s, then perhaps there are further iterations of death to come. Perhaps, doctors will continue to rewrite the rules of human expiration. Disconcertingly, it seems our species possesses mortal fluidity, its definitions of dying in flux over time.

'Pete looks so tired. How long do you think he is going to have to keep doing this?'

I blinked as I listened to Pete's wife, Maria. A frail and elderly woman in her eighties, from the moment she arrived in the hospice she had consistently, unwaveringly, put her husband's needs above her own, despite being terminally ill with renal cancer. Mainly, what gnawed at her was how he would cope without her. Her selflessness moved us all.

'The thing is,' she once confessed, 'all through our marriage he was the breadwinner and I did everything at home.' She paused, then allowed herself a brief, embarrassed smile. 'I'm afraid I'm not certain he could turn on the oven. That probably sounds silly to you.'

'Well, Maria, I'm going to let you into a secret. And it's not one that I'm proud of. On balance, I think I'd prefer it if you didn't tell the nurses.' Her eyes twinkled. I knew she was going to like this. 'I think of myself as a proper, fearless feminist. I would fight tooth and nail for the rights of my daughter – and for all women, everywhere. I can't abide discrimination. But, I have to admit, I am absolutely rubbish at cars. I mean, forget changing tyres, I don't even know how to change the oil in a car. I've literally never done it. Or the water. I leave everything car-related for my husband to sort out. I wouldn't have a clue what to do if I broke down.'

Maria beamed with delight. 'I'd better *not* tell the nurses,' she told me, laughing. 'I don't think they'd be impressed with a doctor here being as hopeless as that.'

Maria and Peter had been married for over fifty years. Their only child died in his infancy. Since then it had been just the two of them, for more than half a century. Every afternoon in the hospice, he sat at her bedside, his knees touching the blankets as he held her hands. It took him two bus journeys to reach the hospital from their home on the edge of the city. Four buses a day, several hours of travelling, with a stick to support his arthritic hip on one side and a hearing aid in his ear on the other. The nurses would bring him tea and cake when he arrived, but he refused all offers of help with transport. I could never discern if it was pride, duty or some other hidden impulse that made him go it alone.

Once we had managed to bring Maria's pain under control, she loved to describe their courting days. 'He was such a catch,' she told me proudly. 'All the girls fancied him, you know.' Throughout the summer, knowing these were likely to be the last months of her life, Maria had taken covert yet decisive action. 'I've filled the freezer with fruit,' she told me. While still strong enough to potter round the fruit farm near their home, she had taken short walks in the sunshine with Pete. It was a bumper season and the freezer shelves soon swelled with strawberries, raspberries and blackberries, carefully apportioned and labelled in tubs and bags for one. An undeclared legacy – the succulence of the summer – waiting to remind him of the woman he loved during these last precious days. 'He won't go hungry this winter,' she said proudly.

It did not stop there. 'The width of fish is a problem,' Maria mentioned one day.

'I'm sorry?' I responded, wondering for a moment if a delirium was brewing.

'Pete doesn't understand that different fish have different widths. Before I came here, I was trying to teach him how to microwave. But a piece of cod will be six minutes, a fillet of plaice only four. It's all there, waiting for him in the freezer, I just don't know if he'll remember that the widths matter.'

That night, I marvelled at this woman so devoted to her husband's well-being that, even while dying of cancer, she had set out to teach him how to survive without her, finding ways to nourish him from beyond the grave, in the bereft and broken days to come. Was there, I wondered, any symbol of love more haunting than this freezer packed from top to bottom with soft fruit and breaded fish?

Now, Maria's most pressing concern was the toll on her husband of his gruelling round trips each day to the hospice. He was visibly exhausted, face taut and grey. Sometimes he looked close to breaking point. I was also aware that her question about how long he must endure the strain was an indirect way of asking for her own prognosis. For a while we talked quietly about how quickly she had changed since arriving here, fatigue first creeping up on her and, latterly, overwhelming her.

She looked me straight in the eye. 'I feel I'm in my last few days,' she told me. 'And I'm not afraid, I'm ready.'

I looked back at her hollow cheeks and shallow breaths. 'I'm so pleased to know you're not afraid, Maria. If that changes, please tell me, we can help.' I paused. 'I think you may well be right about a short number of days. Patients often have a powerful sense of when things are ending, and they're usually right. That's my sense too – that you may well have just days left – and I promise you we will do everything we can to look after you.'

'Just look after Pete,' she instructed me. 'Will you talk to him? Tell him it's close now?'

Following Maria's wishes, that afternoon I invited Pete to have a separate chat. He hovered uncertainly at the foot of her bed, not wanting to leave her. 'Go on, go and talk to her,' she urged him, 'I want you to.'

We sat together in a family room as I gently broached the topic of prognosis. 'Maria suggested we talk about what will happen next,' I said, 'but only if you would feel comfortable doing so. It's completely up to you.'

To my dismay, I saw tears fill his eyes. Early on in palliative medicine, you discover that certain patients are your weakness, the ones whose predicament lances your core. I had always imagined mine would be the mothers of young children – too much identification, too many things shared – but, actually, for me there was something uniquely poignant about elderly men, married for many decades, disintegrating at the prospect of losing their wives. Those masculine tropes of guarding and protecting – how easily cancer undoes them. Even worse is the horrible dawning that, after a lifetime being nurtured domestically, they must somehow survive alone.

For Pete, all of this made facing his wife's death unbearable – a fact she had intuited and for which she had sought my help. But, it turned out, I did not need to be brutally candid. Before I could say anything, his words tumbled out, high-pitched and breathless. 'I can see her going. I know it's coming. I'm losing her. She's going, isn't she?'

I do not know if words exist to comfort a spouse who sees the love of their life sliding away. Perhaps any solace in those moments must be embodied: the physical fact of your presence, sharing the grief in the cord of your own spine. I reached over to close my hand over his and softly squeezed his knuckles. A gasp filled his lungs, sobs caused his shoulders to shudder.

I thought of the fruit – love preserved in freezer-bag form – and whether Pete could ever bear to eat a single morsel. I thought of Dad. It would be like this for us, when the time came. And I experienced a sudden jolt of clarity. That grief is the form love takes when someone dies. That, simply and starkly, the one becomes the other. And that this pain, of all pains, cannot be palliated. Laying bare your heart, to be pulped and flattened, is the necessary price of love.

Once unleashed, Pete's distress seemed to dissipate. He

wanted to know what would happen next. Dying has its own biology, a constellation of signs and symptoms underpinned by our organs shutting down. Choosing my words with care, I began to describe the changes we might see as his wife entered the last phase of her life. There are clues, I explained, that the end is drawing near. Her hands might feel cold as her heartbeat weakened, no longer up to the task of pumping warm blood. We might see her skin become pale, perhaps even slightly blue. Most likely, in the last hours and days, she would slip into deep unconsciousness. Her breathing might become disconcertingly erratic. Deep, shuddering breaths, followed by the longest of pauses in which families often sat on tenterhooks, wondering aghast if another breath would come. *Imagine it, a hundred times through the night – has he just died? No, not quite, not this time, but it is coming.* Some saliva might pool in the back of the throat, I said, unnoticed by Maria but causing a gurgling sound, a rattle, as escaping air bubbled through liquid. This sound can cause more distress among families than any other but rarely, I assured him, are patients aware of it.

Perhaps most reassuringly, I wanted to explain, there is a curious compassion to a person's final days. As they fail, every major organ of the body – our heart, lungs, kidneys, liver – possesses the capacity to anaesthetise the brain, providing the balm of unawareness. Failing lungs lead to the sleepiness of excessive carbon dioxide in the bloodstream. A failing liver or kidneys cause toxins to mount in the blood, blotting and blurring our consciousness. When the blood pressure plummets as an exhausted heart fails, the brain, deprived of its oxygen supply, slows and slides into oblivion. 'It should be gentle,' I told Pete, entirely honestly. 'It is usually gentle, peaceful at the end.'

Whatever the original affliction – cancer, heart failure, cirrhosis, diabetes – in the end, the dying come to resemble each other far more closely than those who, with a similar diagnosis, continue to live. Yet rarely, if ever, is the classical presentation of dying taught at medical school. Small wonder families feel horribly adrift, when even the doctors are ill-equipped to navigate these waters.

As for timescales, I explained, the best guide was what had happened until now. When someone changes over weeks, we suspect they may have an order of weeks to live. If the changes are daily, a lifespan of days is more likely. And when somebody begins to deteriorate hour by hour, then that is the point at which we usually call in a family. The end, we suspect, may be coming in hours.

In Maria's case, her own predictions proved accurate. Several days after asking me to talk to her husband, her renal failure began to cloud the workings of her mind. One morning, this sharp, bright, fearless woman could no longer be roused. The nurses telephoned Pete to tell him she was dying. For once – only this once – he agreed to permit us to send a volunteer driver to collect him. At her bedside he sat, as he had always done, knees to blanket, palm to palm. But this time, while wrapped within the warmth of his hands, Maria's own were cooling and blanching.

The first nine months of Dad's illness comprised the drama of major surgery followed by the endless tedium of chemotherapy. After being sliced wide from sternum to pelvis, he healed remarkably rapidly. He decided there was no time to waste convalescing, walking up and down the length of his ward the day after his surgery. As soon as he recovered, however, he and Mum were forced to adapt to every inch of life being thoroughly hijacked by two unbending dictators, fluorouracil and oxaliplatin. Dad's platinum-based chemotherapy regime proved brutal.

'Nietzsche didn't have a bloody clue,' Dad declared one day. He was referring, I realised, to the crass virility of that famous late-nineteenth-century aphorism 'What does not kill me makes me stronger'.

'I couldn't agree more,' I replied. 'You know that particular bon mot of Nietzsche's was picked as the motto for the Hitler youth camps?'

'Indeed. What utter bollocks.'

The grim truth about chemotherapy, as Dad had swiftly found out, was that each dose of the drugs, loosely targeted at his cancerous cells, was wreaking cumulative havoc on the rest of his body. Worst was the pain in his damaged nerves, raw and shredded from the attentions of platinum. His sense of taste was tarnished for ever, his mouth and skin prone to cracking and bleeding. Fatigue had crept into his bones, sometimes dispatching him to bed for whole days, precious aliquots of life gone for ever. He was weakening, diminishing, week by week, his vitality ebbing away. Mum, my brother, sister and I became ineffectual onlookers, powerless to help him.

I suppose, in one sense, I was lucky. From the moment he was diagnosed, Dad liked to phone me to discuss every nuance of his care, his chances, his options, his prognosis. A doctor adrift on uncharted waters, stripped of the ballast of his old caring role, he needed to analyse it all with a fellow professional he trusted. I could give him that, at least, our long discussions on the phone each night, as soon as I had sorted out the children. I was not entirely impotent. One day, he joked as we chatted, 'Well, all your NHS patients have to share you, Rachel. But I get your undivided attention.'

'Absolutely, Dad. Only platinum-level service for you.'

'Ha! Don't mention the bloody P-word.'

Each time he laughed in our phone calls, afterwards I fought not to cry.

If I gave him anything at all in these conversations, it was small doses of doctorly calm and dispassion, backed up by facts and evidence. By now I was a late-night expert in the management of colorectal cancer, avidly poring over the latest research papers. While we talked, I stamped down hard on the daughter in me – I was damned if I would indulge her. I was fully aware that doctors should never treat anyone close to them, that emotional entanglements risked distorting medical judgements. But in this case I was sounding-board, not decision-maker. I tried to suppress my opinions as ruthlessly as I did my sentimentality. Like all patients, Dad needed to explore and develop his own.

Throughout his chemotherapy, my father floated a pipe-dream. That he might just be one of the statistical outliers, those lucky individuals with aggressive, high-grade, Stage 4 cancer who somehow outlive their doctors' darkest predictions. Everyone always knows an outlier. Usually, they cannot resist regaling a new patient with their uplifting tale of death-defying longevity. Dad himself knew a former NHS nurse, also with Stage 4 colorectal cancer, still going strong a decade after being told she had less than six months to live. If she had done it, he could not help but hope, then so, perhaps, could he. After all, someone, in the end, always won the lottery.

I watched him traverse the ranges of desperation oncology, heart lurching from hope to disappointment as he struggled to weigh the cost of months of chemotherapy against the theoretical chance, however slight, of miraculously beating his statistics. I kept quiet. His opinion was the one that mattered. Each scan, each blood test bludgeoned a little more out of him. After the first three months of chemotherapy, a restaging CT showed it had all been in vain. More cancer, greater spread. The insatiable appetite of those mutant cells. He promptly switched to an alternative cocktail of poisons. Secretly, I wished he had not done so. Then, after another three months on the new regime, the tumour markers in his blood revealed further advancement. He had arrived at the end of the road.

'If I'm honest, I don't think I can face any more chemo,' he told me on the phone that night.

'No,' I agreed. 'It's been a long slog, Dad, hasn't it?'

'I have to say, I'm looking forward to time without it, Rachel.'

At that, I nearly buckled. The attempt to be brave – this determined looking forward – when what he faced, as of today, was the unadorned fact that now there was nothing between him and his cancer. No more delaying or deferring, no clever medical interventions. From this moment forth, his disease would run its natural course. And, as a doctor, he knew all too accurately how this was likely to play out for him. As he spoke, voice unwavering, stripped of all wishful thinking, I had never been more proud of my father.

12

Wonder

How we spend our days is, of course, how we spend our lives.

Annie Dillard, *The Writing Life*

No one is able to inhabit the present quite like those aces of nowness, our children.

Tucked away in a sleepy corner of the London district of Bloomsbury sits a modern-day shrine to children's capacity for wonder. The Foundling Museum tells the story of the Foundling Hospital, Britain's first ever children's charity, established in 1739.

London then was a city teeming with disease, pollution and crippling poverty. Hundreds of babies every year were abandoned by destitute parents across the metropolis – on doorsteps, inside churches, even on rubbish dumps. The deserted infants, the foundlings, often simply died on the street. The aim of the hospital was to provide a home for babies who would otherwise be abandoned, permitting desperate parents to surrender their children, instead, to a place they knew would care for them. Not exactly a hospital, it was more, if you like, a de facto orphanage for infants whose impoverished parents, though very much alive, were no more able to raise them than if buried six feet underground.

Today, the museum works closely with another world-renowned London institution, Great Ormond Street Hospital for Children. The hospital and museum team up periodically to enable young patients to create art installations, which are then exhibited in the museum. The project that captures so beautifully a child's perspective on seizing the day is entitled 'Mead's Mysterious Medicines, 2017'. (Dr Richard Mead – an eighteenth-century physician to royalty and the Foundling Hospital's first doctor – was well known for his restorative potions, whose ingredients he jealously guarded.)

Captivated by the idea of secret elixirs of healing, the museum's artists asked seriously ill children on Great Ormond Street's bone marrow transplant ward to consider the question: If you were to create your own imaginary medicine, what would it contain, and how would it help you? The results are installed on tiny shelves inside the museum. Row upon row of sugar pills in facsimile medicine jars, each meticulously labelled with aims and ingredients. Collectively, they capture the hopes and yearnings of children facing life-threatening diseases, usually cancer. At the time of the project, some of these young patients were certainly old enough to know not only that they might not survive their illness, but also that their only chance of cure was a treatment, a transplant, that in itself was life-threatening.

Shortly after my father decided to abandon chemotherapy, I happened to meander past the Foundling Museum. Unusually, I had a few hours to myself, and although the heat of midsummer drew me to London's streets and parks – the temperature invited basking – I had wanted to visit the museum for years. Forgoing blue skies for air-conditioned sterility seemed, for a moment, a madness.

How wrong I was. On stumbling upon Mead's Mysterious Medicines, I was transfixed. Rooted to the spot before the tiny medicine jars, I avidly read each miniature label. One alone was enough to make my heart clench. Collectively, they were devastating.

'This medicine makes me become a superhero and fly away,' wrote one child. 'Ingredients: Pizza, wings, superheroes, new blood.'

Another wrote: 'This medicine makes it go away. I don't want it. Ingredients: The seaside, stones, the smell of the sea air and seaweed.'

The next bottle was labelled: 'This medicine makes me less sad. Ingredients: Chocolate, my bedroom, mummy, daddy.'

The next: 'This medicine will make me all better. Ingredients: Rainbows, lasagne, orange juice, chocolate milk, art, a meerkat, my two rabbits Clover and Bluebell, milk.'

'This medicine will make me go back home and never come back to hospital. Ingredients: An alien, daddy, my sister Rosie, strawberries, playing in the park, a roast dinner, chocolate pudding and chocolate sauce.'

'This medicine makes the bad luck bones come out of me and the good luck gold go into me. Ingredients: Electricity, a tiger, powerful potions, chocolate, bananas.'

And so it went on.

The bottles were a portal into the wild world we adults used to roam ourselves, in which lasagne and meerkats have magical powers, where milk is as longed for as rainbows, where stones on the shore can obliterate cancer – and where chocolate sometimes trumps even Mummy and Daddy for sheer trans-formational power.

I stood in front of the diminutive jars and found myself whispering their words like an incantation. The loves, fears, hopes and dreams of a wardful of gravely ill boys and girls, distilled within brown glass. It was entirely possible – serious illness being a numbers game, after all – that my own son or daughter might one day inhabit a similar ward, pale and listless, tunnelled lines in their chests, bereft of hair and school and the garden. What spells would they write, how would they fill their bottles? Would Mum and Dad come before or after Finn's homemade slime, Abbey's pet bearded dragon?

Nature looms large in Mead's Mysterious Medicines. Bottled with longing, chosen by children for their power to heal, are: rainbows, rabbits, seaweed, horses' hooves, the woods, laven-der, waves on the beach, summer, the river, the smell of the sea air, raindrops, the outdoors, mint, stones, daffodils, daisies and dew. I imagined the children, trapped in their beds, yet reaching out in their minds beyond the confines of the hospi-tal, breaking out, doing a runner, scattering like marbles along Great Ormond Street, accelerating, high-jumping the M25, then cartwheeling, backflipping in their haste to shed the drips and gowns, to rollick and roll in the grass at last, to sprint head-long into waves, to get on with the serious matters of grazing their knees, peering into rockpools, climbing the nearest trees.

One day, a few weeks after Dad had made his decision to forgo any further chemotherapy, he, Mum and I went for a walk through the fields in which he had happily roamed for nearly forty years. He knew every curve and dip of the land, the smells, the textures, the gifts and surprises. Those spots where, even in midsummer, the ground would be boggy. The glade in which, if you were lucky, you might spot a muntjac. The ditch in which we once temporarily lost the family Labrador as she sank like a stone into ten feet of snow. The tree much favoured by little owls.

That day, Dad's landscape was ablaze with sunshine. I fretted about possible lingering side effects of the chemotherapy that might leave him vulnerable to ferocious sunburn, while he tied his laces and stomped off through the grass, laughing at his doctor-daughter's grumblings about long sleeves and sunhats. Painfully aware his days were numbered, he knew this window of reasonably good health would soon be slammed shut by the cancer. He could have cowered inside, head in hands, imagining cells dividing, invading, overwhelming him. Instead, he tilted his face towards the sky where, reliably, just as I remembered from my childhood, there were skylarks suspended, little loudmouth pinpricks of joy, singing their miniature hearts out. Dad looked outwards and upwards, to the life around him, and it nourished him, even as cancer ate him down, this life going gloriously on.

Can Dennis Potter's concept of 'nowness' – the heightened immediacy of each lived moment – provide solace in the face of death? As someone who cares, every day, for people who are dying, this question is anything but theoretical. Yet I am wary of offering my patients bargain-basement comfort. Unless you have earned the right, like Potter, to speak of dying from experience, how can you be sure your attempts at consolation are not misjudged or, worse, trite and clichéd?

As a newly minted adult, with all the blinkered confidence of youth, I loathed the platitudes and glibness of commercialised self-help. In bookshops, I would cringe at the industrial quantities of paperbacks with titles like *Happiness: Your Route Map to Inner Joy* – though there was, I noted, a pleasing brevity to *Unf*ck Yourself.*

But, towards the tail end of my twenties, it slowly dawned on me that, being an insecure, self-doubting perfectionist myself, I could probably benefit from a little self-help of my own. Chastened, I came up with my own covert strategy for managing anxiety that I privately christened 'the deathbed principle'. As strategies go, it was primitive stuff. After all, its logical extreme was an orgy of unbridled hedonism – not necessarily the best approach for productive living. Nevertheless, when stricken with self-doubt, terrified of failure, I could find perspective by asking myself: 'Would this matter on your deathbed? Seriously, Rach, would you give a damn?'

The great thing, of course, about the view from the shroud is that, from there, almost nothing matters. We all know, deep down, that life's wonder lies in the small stuff. Nobody confronts death thinking, if only the bloody *Lancet* had accepted that paper, if only I'd been knighted, made more money, had more fame. In invoking the deathbed as an insecure young adult, I found I could take the edge off my obsessive high standards and refocus instead upon what, in the end, made life worth living, be it the presence of a loved one, or the sunlight on your cheek, or a palm enclosing yours with warmth.

For Dad, of course, just like my patients, this was no thought experiment. He faced his deathbed for real. Though acutely aware of his own life's brevity, nature brought him unquenchable nowness. Before I specialised in palliative medicine, I had imagined the opposite, that the sheer vitality of nature might be an affront to people so close to the end of life – a kind of impudent abundance, an embarrassment of riches. In fact, in my hospice I am struck by how often, and how intensely, many patients, like Dad, approach the end of their lives finding comfort in the natural world.

One particular patient perplexed us all. A former landscape gardener, his life had been lived in the open air. Now, a furrowed brow and flailing arms were all we had to go on. The indistinct groaning, the way the patient flung his head from side to side – all of it signified an unvoiced anguish. We tried talking, listening, morphine. His agitation only grew.

All cancers have the power to ravage a body, but each assails in distinctive ways. One of the particular cruelties of a cancer of the tongue is its capacity to deprive a person of speech. Some of us thought he must be suffering from terminal agitation, the state of heightened anxiety that sometimes develops as the end of life draws near. But the most junior doctor on the team, Nicholas, was convinced that we could unlock the source of our patient's distress and volunteered to stay behind in the room.

Nicholas reappeared about an hour later. 'You *can* understand his speech,' he announced. 'You just have to really listen.'

When I re-entered the room, the reclining chair that the patient – a tall, angular man in his eighties – had been thrashing around in had been turned to face out on to the garden and the double doors were open wide. Now he sat calmly, transfixed by the trees and sky. All he had wanted was that view.

It is hard to imagine a more potent example of nature's potential to soothe. A growing body of research into the relationship between healthcare and nature points more broadly to the health benefits of opening out hospitals to the natural world or, better yet, finding ways to bring that world inside. In a now classic 1984 paper in the American journal *Science*, the environmental psychologist Roger Ulrich sought to quantify whether being assigned a room with a window view of a natural setting might have 'restorative influences' on a patient.

In 'View through a window may influence recovery from surgery', Ulrich studied the recovery rates of patients who had undergone gallbladder surgery in a suburban Pennsylvania hospital between 1972 and 1981. Patients with bedside windows looking out on leafy trees healed, on average, a day faster than those who saw instead a brick wall, needing fewer painkillers and having fewer post-operative complications.

Even pictures of landscapes may have the power to reduce patients' levels of pain and stress. In a subsequent study in 1993, Ulrich and colleagues randomly assigned 160 heart surgery patients in an intensive care unit to one of six views: simulated 'window views' of a large photograph of a bright, tree-lined stream or a dark forest, one of two abstract paintings, a white panel, or a blank wall. Those patients assigned the water and tree scene were statistically less anxious, and needed fewer doses of painkillers, than those who looked out at the darker forest photograph, the abstract art or no pictures at all. More recent studies demonstrate the benefits of 'distraction therapy', using nature's sights and sounds to reduce the pain and distress of invasive medical procedures such as bronchoscopy. Nature, it seems, is her own elixir.

'There's much talk of being "in the moment", isn't there? Making sure you don't stress out over tiny things that don't matter – so yes, cancer is undeniably a life lesson,' Diane Finch told me wryly. She grinned. 'There's nothing like a diagnosis of secondary breast cancer to pull you up short when you're stressing about having too many dishes to do, for example.'

I first met Diane the day her oncologist broke the devastating news that further palliative chemotherapy – drugs aimed not at cure but at trying to prolong her life – was no longer an option. From this point onwards, her cancer would run its course unimpeded by medicine. 'My first thought, my urge, was to get up and find an open space,' she later explained to me. 'I needed to breathe fresh air, to hear natural noises away from the hospital and its treatment rooms. There is something about being outdoors that trumps anything else. The space, the connection with the sky.'

We were speaking over cups of tea at the bottom of Diane's back garden, a riot of flowers and birdsong. Earlier, in the trees above, some magpies had conducted a guerrilla raid on a nest containing fledgling goldfinches. A few feet away was a tiny pond, recently dug for Diane by her husband, Ed, and their young son, Douglas, which was now, to her delight, overrun with newts. The whole garden, though small, teemed with wildlife.

Diane, fifty-one, had been diagnosed with breast cancer five years earlier. Her son, at the time, was six years old. The hardest blow, she told me, was not the original diagnosis, but the revelation, several years later, that her cancer had returned. 'It's then you realise there's no comeback from it. That's it. You're never going to get rid of it. While it's still a first diagnosis, there's always hope it can be cured, but once it's secondary, it's not curable. Whatever happens to you from now on, the cancer is going to be with you. It is going to be your life partner.'

Diane knew this would be her last summer. Several months earlier, upon discovering her cancer had spread to her brain, she felt a compulsion to try and preserve herself digitally, documenting every thought and feeling on her computer before they, and she, were lost for ever. 'When I had whole brain radiotherapy, I felt like something had dropped out, that I'd lost something. As if everything I said needed to be saved. I'd get this feeling that everything was running away from me, that if I didn't write everything down, somehow I would lose a part of myself.'

But one day, as she was typing frantically, she heard a bird singing through her open window. She paused, transfixed. The experience released her from her frantic efforts at self-preservation. 'Somehow, when I listened to the song of a blackbird in the garden, I found it incredibly calming. I thought, "Well, there will be other blackbirds. Their songs will be pretty similar." And, in the same way, there were other people before me with my diagnosis. Other people will have died in the same way I will die. And it's natural. It's a natural progression. Cancer is part of nature too, and that is something I have to accept, and learn to live and die with.'

Inspired by the blackbird, Diane worked with the hospice music therapist to write her own song, one that, in her words, 'allayed that fear that everything was going to disappear, to be lost for ever'. The act of creation brought her peace.

As we sat and talked on the decking, Douglas's voice now rose from the open window of the kitchen. Clear and light as air, his words were themselves a kind of song. For a moment, Diane stopped and listened. Sorrow tempered the radiance in her eyes. She gathered herself and went on. 'Nature,' she told me, 'is wondrous. It gives us life, it gives us one another, it gives us all these opportunities to love and be loved, it gives us this beautiful world we live in, it gives us the plants and the birds and the animals. It gives us our children. And, of course, cancer is part of nature too. My own body has given me cancer. I have had to accept that I can't have the one without the other. Nature works in cycles, like seasons or waves, and, just as autumn is the winding-down season, well, that is what my life is doing now. I can't control this. None of us can. We have to accept it and do our best to take part with grace, and rejoice in the good things that we've got.'

Diane's equanimity took my breath away. There is the blustering cancer rhetoric of battle and conquest, a vocabulary so many patients loathe – *she's a fighter; she's so brave; if anyone can beat it, she can* – and then there is this: the everyday endeavour to keep grief and fear under wraps while living each day as it comes, as richly as possible, coping, accepting, drawing support from those closest to you, and delighting in the abundance of the world around you. Nature screams from the top of her lungs that everything is fleeting, shifting, disappearing, that nothing lasts, that it is all passing away – and yet, in the words of Gerard Manley Hopkins, 'nature is never spent'. There is also renewal, rebirth, thawing, unfurling. Fledglings, cubs, buds, beginnings. Somehow, Diane's place in these cycles, the planet's rhythms of life, helped still her longing to stop time.

A few weeks after we first met, Diane became my patient. Her room in the hospice seemed permanently filled with sunshine, flowers, people, laughter, cards, presents and, in the periphery, heart-wrenching grief. She was a woman, it was clear, much adored. Her death, when it came, was gentle and communal. Her family sat around her bed until, in the words of her husband Ed, written for her eulogy, 'One morning early in August my son held Diane's hand, and I held his hand, and my sisters held and Steve held and then Diane's hand again. And Diane took just one more breath and that was it. A circle. A chain. And ribbons and skeins of love.'

When I say gentle, I do not mean to convey something false. The absence of pain and distress in Diane's final days may have brought a certain tranquillity to her bedside. But that is not to say, for those who loved her, that her death was not harrowing and dreadful. How could it not be, given how fiercely she was loved? Anguish, as I was learning while my father grew sicker, was the inescapable price of loving. As Ed later put it: 'It's hard, isn't it? A story that starts with us jetting off and crossing continents, climbing mountains and laughing in the face of the storm ends up in a bed in a hospice. With a driver pushing drugs into an arm. A tube carrying away urine. Tiny sips from a straw. Sleep and an end. What a robbery. What a betrayal.'

Later that summer, I would sit among Diane's friends and family as the song she had written was played at her funeral. We heard her voice ring out as truly and exultantly as a blackbird's, and we were spellbound. The lines I loved most of all are these:

Open up your door
There's some birdsong calling
Come on outside
Mr Blackbird says.
Nothing so bad
Can't be improved by choosing
A little light
Instead of the dark.
Steal a little time
Take it back, it's mine
All along the line
A little fresh air.

I looked across the faces around me, at the tears and smiles, pain muddled with delight, and then outside, through the crematorium windows, across fields of wheat, heavy before harvest. Summer was on the cusp of autumn; the world was moving on. And I thought of Philip Larkin's poem 'An Arundel Tomb', whose famous last line has endured since 1956:

'What will survive of us is love.'

A hospice, you might imagine, must be a place overwhelmed by the torment of time running out. How can anyone bear to celebrate the nowness of the moments they have left when each is so close to their last? At its most stark, the answer is simply: in the absence of a choice, you just get on with it, doing the best you can. If that sounds banal, I do my patients a disservice. Their capacity to inhabit the present, in defiance of the future, never fails to astound me.

So, too, did my father's. First, Mum whisked him off on a

romantic minibreak (why should lovesick twentysomethings get all the fun?). They retraced their courting days in the military port of Plymouth – returning to the naval hospital where they first met, the beach where they would sit in their youth, unwrapping fish and chips on the shingle, and the church where they were married, forty-seven years earlier. Nostalgia was twinned with liberation. His life no longer dictated by chemotherapy appointments, Dad revelled in being able to do what he pleased.

'I feel fantastic, Rachel,' he told me one evening. 'I just wish I'd got shot of it sooner. I don't feel sick, I have more energy. It's great.'

Inspired by the success of Plymouth, Dad, being one for bloody-minded extremes, decided to drive his wife all the way to the northwest Highlands of Scotland. Not for a moment did I voice caution. A 1200-mile road trip by a man whose body was beyond even palliative chemotherapy: madness or entirely level-headed? When, in the words of the poet Mary Oliver, life is wild and precious, there is nothing, really, to lose. Dad blithely apportioned what remained of his to a place that incites unruly living, the hunch-backed, knife-edged mountains of Torridon.

The sandstone peaks of this glacial landscape are among the oldest and most spectacular summits in Britain. When I was a child, Dad led me up the pinnacles of Liathach, golden eagles above, sheer walls of rock falling away below. One false move, one misplaced boot, and you could smash your reckless brains out. I discovered the strange exhilaration of traversing a landscape that was supremely indifferent to your life in its grasp. When I finally stood with Dad on the summit, elated and trembling, I felt almost drunk on my own inconsequentiality. Up here, we were nothing, not even dust in the wind. The world had never felt larger.

Over the years, Dad kept returning to Torridon. The wildness seduced him. On this trip, any actual ascent was, of course, out of the question. Even a stroll was a major exertion. It did not matter. He stood with his wife in the foothills and scaled every summit in his mind, feasted on their sandstone skirts, thrilled at the sight of a sea eagle. Not just any eagle, of course, but the final eagle. The final mountain. The final Scottish langoustines, drenched in garlic butter. The final glimpse of heather, granite, red deer and quartz. Without a shred of self-pity, he devoured every moment.

Back home, we found a new rhythm. Every Wednesday, the moment my work on the ward was complete I would claw my way westwards through motorway gridlock to arrive, at last, at the family home for a night and a day with my parents. On the doorstep, Dad would embrace me tightly, his vertebrae jutting like flints through his shirt. Covertly, I would appraise the week's weight loss. Mum would have carefully concocted a meal for two and a half, hoping to entice her husband into grazing. He still enjoyed fish, the odd omelette and cheese, eating partly for himself, but mainly for our benefit. He was well aware that his growing fatigue was a consequence of cancer, not loss of appetite. What multiplied inside him was voracious for fuel, first the fat, then the muscle, that vanished from Dad's bones. My finger and thumb could encircle his wrist. His clothes hung like sheets from a line.

For all his gauntness and increasing lethargy, Dad's spirits were remarkably buoyant. We laughed and raged about the forty-fifth President and argued, as ever, about Brexit. He nearly made me drop the teapot one morning, so loudly did he yell 'Sparrowhawk!' from behind the kitchen sink, gesticulating frantically at the small brown shape scything across the garden. He stopped needing to dissect every detail of his health. Nothing was at stake now, none of it mattered. He wisely refused further scans and blood tests. Better not to enquire too closely about the upheavals and dissolution within. Better instead to focus on what made him feel human. Temporarily absolved from being Dad's ad hoc doctor, I reassumed with gratitude the role of daughter.

One crisp Sunday afternoon, after a hastily snatched weekend with my parents, Dad drove me back to the train station. Perhaps it was fatigue, perhaps his mind was simply elsewhere, but as he approached an urban roundabout, he accidentally pulled out in front of a motorbike. There was no slamming of brakes, no screech of rubber on tarmac. No one's adrenalin surged. Nevertheless, the rider decided to pursue us all the way to the station, tailgating the car and aggressively revving the throttle. As soon as Dad parked up, the man was there, all six foot plus of him, slamming his fists on the windscreen and hurling abuse at my father.

Dad eased his skeletal legs out of his seat, wincing as he raised himself to standing. Oblivious to his frailty, and to his repeated apologies, the man's torrent of abuse only escalated.

'You fucking prick. You fucking moron. What the fuck do you think you're playing at?'

A finger jabbed the air, closer and closer to Dad's face, the moment crackling with the nearness of physical violence. Stooped and submissive in the face of this invective, my father looked painfully vulnerable. Appalled, I stepped between him and his assailant, forcing him to turn instead to me.

'What do you think you're doing? Stop attacking my dad. He's said sorry. Listen to him. He's already said sorry. What more do you want? If you're going to hit someone, hit me. Don't hit an old guy. Hit me if that will make you feel better.'

It was rash, foolish and wholly impulsive. The man's fists were raised and he towered over me. But in that moment, my instinct to protect my father was as fierce as any towards my children. It was all I could do to stop myself from screaming: 'He's dying of cancer! Do you understand? He's *dying*. Do you really have to make things any worse?'

The man spat on the ground and roared off on his bike as my train pulled into the station. Dad ushered me off, assuring me he was fine, and I ran for the nearest carriage. Once seated, I could not stop shaking. The aggression, the snarling, every moment had been awful. But what lingered as the country-side streaked past my window, an undulating riptide of blue and green, was the realisation that this role reversal was final. Father, colossus, bedrock, sage. All my life, in all the dramas big and small, Dad had known what to do. From blocked sinks to flat tyres, from my own cancer scare to Finn's harrowing first days in a neonatal ITU, Dad had been there, guiding and protecting me. Now, both psychologically and physically, he was the one needing me.

A decade before he knew he was dying, my father and I made a death pact. The deal we struck was that, once medically qualified, I would access the morphine with which to assist him in ending his life, should he be diagnosed with something unbearable.

'I couldn't stand being a vegetable, Rachel,' he told me. 'If I'm going gaga with dementia, or I have a catastrophic stroke or something, I want you to put me out of my misery.'

'I will, Dad. Don't worry. I will.'

This response, I should stress, was as glib as it was probably dishonest. What I actually thought, though kept unvoiced, was that should such an appalling set of circumstances present themselves, well, then I would be forced to evaluate them. But, at the time, I saw no benefit in refusing to give my father the reassurances he wished for. A sense of mortal control, via the pledges of his daughter, seemed to help him confront his old age.

The death vows were renewed on a regular basis. Dad had a deep, festering fear of losing his dignity in the fog of a disease like dementia. He liked to reconfirm on a regular basis that, should the time come, I would do what was necessary. I never questioned the ethics of potentially lying to my father. Like his promises, years ago, to the dying naval ratings with full-thickness burns, I believed I was giving him necessary comfort, while suspecting I could never do what he asked of me. I was acting, first and foremost, as a daughter, not a doctor.

At work one day in the hospice, I realised that, ever since being diagnosed with cancer, Dad had not mentioned assisted dying. Of all the times you might think it would matter – when confronting the abyss, actual terminal cancer – he saw no need to resurrect that conversation. And this was not, I believed, because he had unwavering faith in me reaching for the fatal doses of morphine, if necessary. It was the opposite: he no longer seemed to have need of them. His acceptance of death allowed him simply to live, savouring the moments left to him.

But what of those patients so terrified of dying they can

think of nothing else? Where acceptance is out of the question, so ghastly is the existential dread that consumes them? Philip Larkin's poem 'Aubade' is, perhaps, the greatest depiction of thanatophobia, or anxiety caused by thoughts of one's death. An aubade is traditionally a song or poem that joyously heralds the dawn, usually involving lovers parting at first light. But Larkin's aubade, written in 1977, is bleak and ironic, describing the poet waking to 'soundless dark' after a night's heavy drinking. Paralytic with fear, he waits for dawn to break, horribly aware that:

> *Till then I see what's really always there:*
> *Unresting death, a whole day nearer now*

This prospect, for Larkin, is so appalling that his 'mind blanks at the glare'. Nothing can bring him solace, neither the tricks of religion nor the specious argument that it is irrational to fear something which, by definition, you will never feel. This, Larkin argues, is precisely the point: for what could be ghastlier than your own obliteration? He spells out the horror for us:

> *. . . this is what we fear – no sight, no sound,*
> *No touch or taste or smell, nothing to think with,*
> *Nothing to love or link with,*
> *The anaesthetic from which none come round.*

Exceptionally rarely, I encounter dying patients who, like Larkin, are so haunted by the prospect of their imminent death that nothing is capable of bestowing comfort or consolation. The act of living, as death bears down, is a harrowing psychological ordeal. If a patient is suffering desperate, intractable distress in the last hours or days of their life, a treatment option of last resort – for when symptoms cannot be relieved by any other means – is that of 'continuous deep sedation'. The patient is freed from their anguish when sedatives are administered to the point of unconsciousness.

Continuous deep sedation is crucially different from assisted dying and euthanasia since its aim is not to hasten death but, instead, to relieve suffering. The vast majority of patients do not require such drastic measures. Usually, low doses of sedating medications are sufficient to soothe a person's fears, while allowing them still to interact with their loved ones and the world around them.

Paradoxically, in palliative medicine there is also the other extreme: patients who have suffered crippling thanatophobia throughout their life, yet for whom a terminal diagnosis is essentially curative. Once, I cared for a man whose prostate cancer had spread throughout his skeleton, causing multiple fractures in his legs and spine. Roger arrived at the hospice in severe pain, paralysed from the waist down, having been told he was in the last days or short weeks of his life. But when I met him, he was grinning so broadly I wondered whether I had entered the wrong room.

As we talked over the coming days, he painted a picture of a lifetime's anguish. 'I first thought about suicide when I was a child, Rachel. I know that sounds ridiculous, in the context of being so frightened of dying, but the thought of being nothing, of just ceasing to be, made me sick with dread. The pointlessness of life. Why go on? Why live another day of pain when it's all so utterly futile?'

Roger, now in his fifties, had suffered intermittently from severe anxiety and depression all his life, with multiple psychiatric admissions to hospital. 'I know Freud would say my fear of death is really a fear of something else, some unresolved childhood conflict or other, but he's wrong. I can remember my skin crawling, even as a kid, at realising that all human life must end, including mine.'

'So what's going on now, Roger?' I asked him. 'Forgive me, but you're in a hospice and yet you seem so . . . happy.'

'Yes. Yes, I am. I can honestly say that being told I'm dying is the best thing that's ever happened to me.'

We both burst out laughing. It was true. Once we had managed to sort out his pain, Roger's demeanour was that of a college student on spring break. 'I feel free,' he said. 'This is the first time in my life I've ever felt relaxed. Isn't that bizarre? None of my fears bother me any more. All the things like the kindness of the nurses, a massage in the morning, time with my family – I can just enjoy them without worrying. It's beautiful.'

For the last two weeks of his life, Roger was liberated from a lifetime's angst. He knew, for the first and only time, what it was to be at peace. Death, it turned out, was not what released him but, rather, his knowledge of its imminence.

13

The Man with the Broken Heart

I don't understand how the last card
is played,
But somehow the vital connection is made.

Elastica, 'Connection'

It is Friday night in the emergency department, not yet the bedlam of pub closing time, but already the atmosphere is charged and bristling. Someone drunkenly chants football songs in one corner, clutching a blood-soaked clump of paper towels to his scalp wound. A few chairs down, a young woman shouts abuse at her partner. In the main waiting area, which has run out of seats as usual, the eight-hour wait to be seen is written all over the faces, strained and angry, of people close to breaking point.

To me, it is all background noise. My focus is the man behind the curtain I am about to draw, my next patient, who appears enigmatically on the computers in Majors only as 'Male – pacemaker problems'.

I am intrigued. A pacemaker is a wonder of modern medicine. A tiny device the size of a matchbox, it consists of a generator, a battery and two wires known as pacing leads. The whole thing is surgically embedded beneath the skin of the chest, just below the left collarbone. Each pacing lead is guided through a blood vessel into the heart itself, where they sit, often for years, poised to send waves of electricity up and down the heart, when required, to stimulate normal beating.

Cardiac electrophysiology is nail-biting stuff. Those sixty or seventy heartbeats per minute – two billion beats over the course of a lifetime – are ordinarily triggered by the heart's own, inbuilt pacemaker, a group of cells some five millimetres wide that generates the electrical flow behind each cardiac contraction. Imagine a kettle or smartphone or car or computer maintaining that kind of output, without glitch or malfunction, for a solid eight or nine decades. Evolution beats engineering hands down. But, should a disease trigger an electrical storm – the heart beating too quickly, slowly or erratically to maintain someone's blood pressure – then the patient may collapse without warning or, worse, suffer a cardiac arrest. The engineers' backstop, this matchbox of tricks, is an ingenious fix for what might otherwise be fatal cardiac arrhythmias.

I am hoping my patient will have a dramatic ECG, a trace of something rare on the print-out or even, if I am lucky, a heart condition I have never seen before. I feel vaguely guilty at my eagerness to meet him.

Mr Richardson – Michael, as he permits me to call him – has his thin, bony arms folded protectively around his chest. It is almost as though he has something to hide. He has the furtiveness of a teenaged girl, ashamed of the new contours into which her body has erupted. Michael, however, is in his late eighties. He looks thoroughly miserable and desperate to leave. I smile warmly as I introduce myself, hoping to put him at ease.

'I know I should have come here sooner,' he begins, before trailing away into awkward silence, staring down at the floor.

'That doesn't matter,' I reassure him. 'The important thing is that you're here now.'

He looks up with no less anxiety. 'Did the nurses tell you what the problem is?'

'No, but whatever it is, we're here to help. That's all that matters.' His face looks flushed and I wonder about infection as I wait for him to continue.

'Well,' he says uncertainly, starting to uncross his arms, 'the problem is this thing here.'

As his gown slides away with theatrical suspense, it is the smell that accosts me first, the reek of putrefaction. And there, to my horror, gingerly cradled in both his hands, is his pacemaker, slithering in blood and pus, dangling from a hole in his chest. My first instinct – more visceral than medical – is to shove the thing back inside. I want to tug the skin back together, suture it shut, cover up the crater where intact flesh should be.

Michael looks contrite and embarrassed. 'I know I should have come here sooner,' he says again. 'Do you think you'll be able to fix it so I can go home this evening?'

'Well,' I say calmly, 'one step at a time. Don't worry, we will be able to sort this out, but perhaps not overnight. Tell me, how did it begin?'

In A&E, you must be adept at inscrutability. The exclamations you yearn to blurt – *How many times? MI5 made you do it? You say you sat on an . . . artichoke?* – must be instantly transformed into bland, polite, innocuous enquiries that give away not a hint of prurience. In this case, the question I long to ask is: 'How, in the name of all that lives, could you possibly have left this infection in your chest to deepen and spread and entrench and fester until – bam – it exploded like a rotten melon? How could you not have sought help sooner?'

But things are rarely as simple as they first seem in a hospital and, sure enough, the story that emerges is the furthest thing from inexplicable. A few weeks ago, Michael had visited hospital to have the battery in his pacemaker replaced. A simple procedure, performed under sterile conditions and local anaesthetic, it should have been a formality. Unluckily for Michael, during the unzipping, burrowing and restitching of his chest, conditions were less than aseptic. After a few days he began to notice redness and pain at the site of his stitches, but ignored them, hoping they would disappear. The more his chest wall throbbed, the more it swelled and reddened, the more certain he was that he needed medical assistance. This was, after all, a human heart we were talking about. Infection of a device whose wires were tunnelled directly inside those beating chambers was clearly not to be ignored.

But something meant more to Michael than his own heart – that of his wife of fifty years. Ever since Mary had been diagnosed with dementia three years earlier, he had been her sole carer. He cooked for her, dressed her, bathed her and soothed her. When she cried because she could not remember the name of her sister, Michael was the one who could make her smile. He knew she liked warm milk and honey at bedtime. He remembered that stroking her arm could quell a rising panic. If he went into hospital, who would care for Mary?

Terrified that his wife might end up in a care home without him, Michael had ignored the pain in his chest for as long as was humanly possible. Then, this morning, as he reached for a plate from a cupboard, he had felt the skin rip apart. Suddenly, his shirt was drenched in thick pus. The infection that had smouldered for weeks inside his chest had caused the scar above his pacemaker to burst apart, exposing ribs and lungs to daylight. Only then, while clutching a matted knot of blood and wires, did he concede defeat and call the paramedics.

As Michael told me this story, his shoulders sagged and he began to cry. Exactly as he had feared, Mary had been whisked away by social services to an emergency care home for her own protection. There were no other family or friends to care for her. She could not have survived at home on her own. Now, Michael knew, she was alone, confused, abandoned and frightened, while he, quite literally, was broken-hearted.

I sat down on the bed beside him and took his hand. 'Tell me about Mary,' I said gently. 'How did you two first meet?'

He squeezed my fingers as he began to depict the vivacious young woman who liked dances, the seaside and whisky and ginger. I knew the cardiologists could sort out a new pacemaker and that with luck, in a few days' time, intravenous antibiotics would get him well. But I also sensed that his extraordinary efforts to keep his wife by his side had been growing increasingly desperate. His grief, in part, was for the fragile home he had fought so hard to preserve but which now, perhaps, was irrevocably shattered.

'Michael, you have done an astonishing job of keeping Mary at home with you,' I said. 'What an act of love it has been. You are a truly exceptional husband.'

I hoped my words might give him some small solace, but there was no softening his anguish. Bereft and sobbing, he turned to the wall as I went to call the cardiologists.

On that frenetic Friday in A&E, I longed to believe that Michael and Mary would be reunited in a shared home in a residential community, sufficiently supported to spend their remaining days together, which was all that mattered to them. Given our threadbare, underfunded social services, I knew that the image was almost certainly a pipedream. But what stood as an incontrovertible fact – a testament to human goodness – was that on this day I met a man who so loved his wife of sixty years that he sacrificed his heart for hers. And, in the end, when death bears down, there is always this, the love of others. Greater than nowness, greater than nature, greater than moments of sensory pleasure: the power of human connection.

Sometimes I wonder whether, had Philip Larkin known more of what happens to patients after they die in a hospice, he might have felt a little less haunted by the aloneness of death. As an atheist, I have no heavenly consolation, but my patients' immediate afterlife on earth can have a transcendence all of its own. As so often, in life as well as death, some of the most extraordinary human connections in the hospice are those forged by the nurses.

Shortly after I started working with Nina, we began chatting about how she tended to her patients after death. This was not your average conversation, corpses, after all, tending to provoke revulsion. But for us, our patients are still our patients, even after an illness has claimed them. The care does not stop with the heartbeat. Recently, the whole hospice had been rocked by the death of a patient far too young to die.

'It must be one of the hardest things, mustn't it, as a parent?' said Nina. 'To lose your child when it should be you who goes first.'

'Yes,' I agreed. 'I honestly believe I would sacrifice my life if it kept Finn and Abbey alive. I can't imagine the heartbreak of losing your children.'

Toby, the man we were discussing, was scarcely more than a child himself when he died of a rare degenerative neurological disorder, at only nineteen. Throughout the final two weeks of his life his mother, Jackie, was by his side in the hospice night and day. Too weak to stand and reach a commode or bathroom, Toby had been forced to surrender his dignity to his nurses who kept him clean and comfortable. For any patient, this can be profoundly traumatic, but for a man so young, barely across the cusp of adulthood, the dependence on others was mortifying.

The bond that Nina developed with Toby was forged, in part, through gentle tactility. It was Nina, one evening, who inserted the catheter so his urine could collect into a bag, preserving him from the humiliation of wetting himself. It was Nina who changed his sheets and pyjamas when he developed diarrhoea. And it was Nina who held his hand in the early hours of the morning, when Toby's panic threatened to overwhelm him and he fought not to cry in front of his mother. Nina witnessed, respected and never flinched from his pain. Nor his sobbing. Nor his fear. Nor his bodily fluids. For twelve-hour shifts at a time. Invariably, she managed to make him smile. She even tried, at his insistence, to play a game on his Xbox, though his verdict, as he wiped away tears of laughter, was: 'Lady, stick to nursing.'

It was Nina's touch, more than anything, that seemed to still

Toby's fears and, immediately after he died, it was her touch again that framed his life after death for Toby's grieving family.

'It matters, doesn't it?' she told me. 'Those last days, those last hours, that's what a loved one is never going to forget. So, we always make sure it's nice for them. A dab of something nice and scented behind the patient's ears, really good mouth care, keeping the teeth and tongue clean. That really matters. The smell, you see. It needs to be clean, not horrible, or families will always remember a nasty smell of death. You don't want to leave them with that in their heads.'

Seated in Toby's room, at the moment of his death, were his brother, sister, father and mother. They had sat vigil, round the clock, for twenty-four hours as Toby's breathing stuttered and faltered. At the final breath – the lingering pause that slowly, subtly, revealed itself to be not a pause but an ending – Nina was there too, keeping watch on him and his family. When the storm of tears had subsided, she suggested she might wash Toby's body. Everyone left the room apart from Jackie. Together, the two women, nurse and mother, undressed and soaped and sponged his body.

'I don't know how to do this,' Jackie said to Nina.

'Just like this. See, nice and gentle. We can get him all clean and fresh together.'

Nina's guidance was deft and respectful, allowing Jackie to feel she was every inch a mother. 'This is me showing my son I love him,' Jackie whispered. 'Thank you. I didn't realise I could do this.'

After the rest of the family returned, Toby's sister noticed his stubble. 'What about his face, Mum? He hated not being properly shaved.'

And so, on Nina's expert lead, a mother and a seventeen-year-old sister lathered Toby's pale cheeks and tenderly began to shave him. Even after death, he was son, brother, human.

'I won't ever forget this,' Toby's sister said to Nina, razor in hand. 'I never knew this is what you did for someone after they died.' Then, she turned to her brother. 'I love you, Toby. I will always love you.'

When doctors forget to treat patients as people, terrible acts can result. As I write, the British press is full of shocking headlines concerning an eminent liver transplant surgeon, Simon Bramhall, who recently pleaded guilty to branding his initials upon the livers of two separate patients. As they lay unaware, anaesthetised and opened wide on his operating table, Bramhall used an argon beam coagulator, conventionally deployed to stop intraoperative bleeding, to burn the letters 'S B' into his patients' organs.

'It was an intentional application of unlawful force to a patient whilst anaesthetised,' stated Elizabeth Reid, of the Crown Prosecution Service, during his criminal trial. 'His acts in marking the livers of those patients, in a wholly unnecessary way, were deliberate and conscious acts on his part.'

The case provoked widespread, though not universal, condemnation. Several patients whose lives Bramhall had saved with a liver transplant leapt publicly to his defence. The majority of reactions, however, from both inside and outside the medical profession, ranged from consternation to revulsion. Though the brandings did not, reportedly, cause any physical harm, there is a chilling arrogance to an act whose subtext is: 'You're mine. Your body is at my disposal and I can do whatever I like to it.' As Joyce Robins, a spokesperson for the charity Patient Concern, commented, 'This is a patient we are talking about, not an autograph book.'

How can a doctor possibly think it is acceptable to brand their patients like cattle? The case is even more extraordinary when you consider that Bramhall did not have a reputation as a monster. By all accounts he was a skilful and even compassionate surgeon who had an excellent rapport with his patients. Perhaps though, for as long as the medical profession continues to expect its own to suppress their feelings, disguise their distress and fake bravado, it risks breeding warped attitudes from doctors towards patients.

Too often, a stiff upper lip in the face of human anguish is expected from day one. I think of my friend Tom, twenty-six, an intensive care doctor, who told me one morning of the night he had spent fighting to stabilise a young woman on his ITU. The same age as him, she was mown down by a car on a zebra crossing, causing severe back, neck and head injuries. In the morning handover meeting, the day team assembled in crisp blue scrubs to briefly dissect the events of the night. The lead consultant surveyed the dying young woman's charts: 'Well, your nocturnal efforts were a waste of time, weren't they, Tom? Couldn't you see it was futile?'

The obliteration of young life, and its casual dismissal, caused Tom to do something unexpected. He found his eyes were filling with tears. For the rest of the handover, as they spilled down his face, not one doctor or nurse in the crowded room found it in themselves to acknowledge his distress. They pretended they had not seen it.

Occasionally, in the hospice, keeping company with the

dying can feel overwhelming. On a bad day there are moments when the weight of the sadness is almost palpable, the air so thick with grief and loss that I feel I am inhaling pure pain. But I am lucky. I work on a ward where, if I have just spent an hour talking to a father and his children about the fact that their mother is dying, I may return to my computer to find someone has quietly placed a cup of tea and some biscuits beside it. We seek each other out, we get through it together. These small acts of solidarity – a hug, a Custard Cream, the offer of a quiet chat – ensure no one shoulders their bad days alone. Vital connections, human to human, can mean so much to our patients. It would be strange if we neglected them among ourselves.

As my father grew weaker, I found myself working harder and harder. I desperately wanted every one of my patients' deaths to be, at the very least, gentle. Preferably, they should all be preceded by last weeks and days that thrummed with life. I knew perfectly well what I was doing, attempting to offset my dread of what I knew was looming by trying to prove to myself that it could be beautiful, joyous – even right at the end. If I could store up enough examples of dying without anguish, then perhaps I could stand it when Dad died.

One morning, a text came from Mum. 'Call me,' it said. 'Dad is in pain.' The hairs on my neck tingled with foreboding. Explaining my absence to my colleagues, I rushed outside to call her back.

'He's not well,' Mum said hastily. 'He's had to take morphine. And it's not working. Speak to him, he wants to speak to you.'

Dad came on to the line, apologetic, slightly muddled, muttering about not wanting to disturb me at work.

'Dad,' I said, 'please don't worry about that. Now tell me what's happening.'

Whether it was morphine, pain or fear I could not tell, but Dad's precise and technical medical vocabulary had blurred into confused incoherence. Piece by piece, a picture formed. It was his liver, I was certain, that wracked his body with spasms. The flesh was being painfully stretched by the burgeoning weight of his liver metastases.

'Dad, please take more morphine. You've nothing to lose when you're in this much pain. Just get on top of it and then we can plan. I'm going to ask Mum to call your GP out. Steroids might help. But let's get you assessed properly.'

Every illness trajectory is unpredictable. I am, for example, currently caring for a man who was diagnosed with six months to live from his cancer – twenty years ago. But in this moment with Dad, I was horribly certain that the end, at last, was beginning.

I walked unsteadily back on to the ward to see Laurie, the ward sister. 'I'm sorry,' I blurted. 'I don't think I can work any more. It's Dad. I – I think this is it for him. He's got awful liver capsular pain and he sounds encephalopathic. I just don't think I can see any more patients.'

She made me feel like I was not a quitter, but a sensible doctor who recognised her limits. She told me I was putting my patients first, when I believed I was failing them. My bosses at work could not have been kinder. They told me to go, to be there for my father, even though they would have to shoulder my absence. I walked out of the hospice into crisp winter sunshine. Consumed by guilt, grief and trepidation, I knew the next death I would witness would be my father's.

14

Gratitude

*What are we here for if not to enjoy life eternal, solve what problems
we can, give light, peace and joy to our fellow-man, and leave this
dear fucked-up planet a little healthier than when we were born?*

Henry Miller, *This Is Henry, Henry Miller from Brooklyn*

The first thing I see, on arriving back home, is how skil-
fully and gently Mum has resurrected her nurse's role. It is as
though she has, of necessity, expanded, filling the space around
Dad, who is shrinking. Somehow, through a thousand subtle
acts of daily care, she is managing, without making him feel
diminished or unmanned, to attend to all his needs, including
those he is unaware of. The hollows beneath her eyes, darkly
smudged with exhaustion, alarm me. She barely sleeps. This
cannot be sustainable. But nothing will deny her these last acts
of love, least of all the limits of stamina.

As for Dad, behind his smile I see a new apprehension in his
eyes. When this new pain ambushed him, he knew, like me,
exactly what it signified. *Here we are, Mark. We've arrived at the*

endgame. 'This is it,' I knew my father was thinking. 'How bad is it going to be?'

Mum gives me a meaningful stare. Dad's jaundice is severe now, his eyes and skin stained darkest yellow. I saw how slowly he shuffled to the front door just now. *Oh, Dad.* Everything inside is starting to disintegrate and there is absolutely nothing we can do about it.

We gingerly embrace. His bones, stripped of flesh, cannot take any pressure. But as we kiss, his eyes light up. Of course. It is a Wednesday. '*Peaky Blinders* tonight, Rachel.' Dad is addicted to the BBC television series depicting gang warfare on the mean streets of 1920s Birmingham and, in solidarity, I have started watching too.

'I know, right? Want to have a bet on how many corpses we'll have by the end of the episode?'

'More than that,' Dad replies. 'I want to know if you've got to the bottom of the milk people. Have you? It's been playing on my mind.'

I laugh. Early on in Donald Trump's presidency, a transcript emerged of a telephone exchange with Malcolm Turnbull, the Australian Prime Minister, which included a mysterious reference to America's 'local milk people'. Social and mainstream media descended into frenzied speculation as to who or what, exactly, Trump's milk people were. The phrase became a viral meme and Dad, like the rest of the world, had loved coming up with absurd possibilities.

'Well, I'm very concerned about the milk people too, Dad. Even the *Washington Post* hasn't figured out who they are yet. Honestly, I know you've got cancer but, really, there are bigger issues out there, you know.'

Dad chuckles as he returns to his favourite chair, straight-backed, well-upholstered, with strong wooden arms he can lean on to haul his skeletal frame to standing.

'You two sit and chat,' says Mum. 'Wine, Rachel?'

'Most definitely,' I reply.

My familiarity with patients in their final days, the various contours and derangements of dying, have prepared me not a jot for the shock of seeing Dad among their number. It is perfectly clear time is short now. *This is it. How bad is it going to be?*

After Mum discreetly disappears to the kitchen, we stop joking. Quietly, I ask him straight out: 'How are you really feeling, Dad?'

His smile, in response, is bittersweet. For a moment, neither one of us speaks. With absolute clarity we both can see that his dying has taken on an irresistible momentum.

I am reminded of the character in Ernest Hemingway's *The Sun Also Rises* who, when asked how he went bankrupt, answers, 'Gradually and then suddenly.' Dad's dying is the bankruptcy kind – a long stealthy creep, then the precipitous fall. He is teetering on the cliff edge, and he knows it. That smile, more than anything, was one of mutual recognition. From doctor to doctor, it is all understood. No need to discuss what comes next.

A stab of self-doubt rushes through me. We may be doctor and doctor, and also doctor and patient, but we are father and daughter, too. I am being stretched impossibly thinly. My heart feels like it may rupture.

'The pain is quite bad,' Dad admits.

I focus. The daughter will just have to wait. We start calmly discussing his symptoms. It turns out that Dad is well aware he should take more morphine, but something ill-defined, yet potent, is holding him back. Like many patients, he has imbued the drug with symbolic finality. In his mind, this is no mere analgesic, a paracetamol or codeine, it is the end of the line, an elixir of doom. Morphine is the death drug, the last breath drawing near. One sip, and you may as well have downed cyanide.

'I know what you mean, Dad, and I think I might feel the same. But logically, it's just a painkiller. It doesn't signify anything, except in Victorian novels, but it does get the job done. Why don't you experiment? Put up the dose a bit, see if it helps? If you feel sleepy or sedated, you can just take it down again. This time is precious and it's hard to enjoy anything if you're hurting.'

To my surprise, Dad agrees immediately. 'He trusts you,' Mum says later. 'He feels safe when you're here.'

That night, the three of us sit in front of the television and watch *Peaky Blinders*. A bit of torture, a corpse or two, something awful involving a vat of red paint, the famously wandering Birmingham accents. Dad's extra dose of morphine has eased the gnawing in his liver. He laughs, interacts, nods off once or twice, reawakens. It is a perfect ordinary family evening, replicated in a million homes across the country, with an added dash of terminal cancer. And, really, it could not be lovelier. No angst, no anguish, just two parents and their daughter, enjoying the easy warmth of the sofa.

Ever a creature of habit, Dad adopts a daily routine. Too weak to stand for long now, in the mornings he sits to brush his teeth, while I assemble his drugs for him. Then, I carefully accompany him downstairs, acutely aware that, any day now, this descent will be too much for him. Sitting in his favourite chair, he tries a mouthful of Weetabix, a few sips of water, and makes a start on the newspaper. The print often swims, the effort of reading makes him drowsy, but always, without fail, he finds something that requires animated discussion. I remember why, as a nine-year-old who liked gymnastics, I had surprisingly strong views on the English cricketer Ian Botham.

Three times a day, Mum rubs soothing cream into the points along her husband's body where the skin, stretched taut as wire across ridges of bone, is at risk of breaking down. The gentle massage is more than a nurse's expert care, it is love that she transmits through her fingertips. In the afternoons, Dad rests in bed now, sometimes all the way into the evening. Sleepier and sleepier with each passing day, he is enacting the very conversation I have held so many times before, explaining to frightened men and women the classical patterns of dying. Everything is as he had hoped. He is at home, not in hospital, surrounded by his wife and children, his grandchildren visiting as often as school allows. There is little pain and only occasional confusion. I should be grateful and, really, I am. But soon, so soon, his sleep will be ceaseless. At night, I lie awake in silent tears. *Dad, oh Dad, I can't bear to lose you.*

Bit by bit, over fifteen long months, cancer has stolen from my father just about all it is possible to cull from a body. Soon he will be too weak even to rise from his bed. Yet his spirit and good humour endure. About a week before the end, his wristwatch stops at night while he sleeps. 'Well that's just marvellous,' he tells me wryly, in the morning. 'Talk about being told your time is up.'

Later that day, I ask him, 'Are you scared of dying?'

He smiles. 'Of dying? No, not of that. Of symptoms, maybe. But my only regret is that I will never see my grandchildren grow up into adults. I have lived a wonderful life.' It seems perverse to describe a dying man as lucky, but all I can think in this moment is that here, surely, is the very definition of being blessed.

In the small hours of sleeplessness, I ponder Dad's equanimity. In the end, for him, like so many of my patients, it is biography, not biology, that matters. He has been spared the distress of pain and other harrowing symptoms. His body, as it slowly disengages from the world, does so with surprising placidity. Thrust to the forefront of his mind, therefore, is the narrative thread of his life. The job that meant so much to him, his three young grandchildren, the wife he has loved for nearly half a century, the children he raised and who now draw close, like moths to his flame, to support and care for their father. In this living legacy, spanning three generations, he finds the deepest fulfilment.

'Be kind while you can,' he tells me. I am half sitting, half lying on his bed beside him. He has just woken up after spending most of the day sleeping.

Before I can stop myself, I find myself sobbing, childishly, frantically. 'I don't want you to die, Dad.'

He smiles and places my hand on my chest, enveloped in his. He presses down. 'Rachel,' he says, 'you know I won't be gone. I will keep living in here, and in Finn, and in Abbey.'

I nod as I try to compose myself. I know he is referring to the only afterlife that counts.

'All those crazy Silicon Valley billionaires who keep coming up with technology to try and live for ever, they've so missed the point, haven't they, Dad?' I say.

He laughs. 'They certainly have. The only immortality that matters to me is knowing my family and friends might still think of me occasionally.'

'We will, Dad. You know we will.'

He does not answer. He has drifted off to sleep again. But he knows it.

In an attempt to salve my anticipatory grief, at night I read a collection of essays by the late neurologist and author Oliver Sacks. Published posthumously and written shortly after his own diagnosis of terminal cancer, Sacks' final thoughts, on looking back over eight decades of living and loving, are overwhelmingly those of thankfulness. Entitled *Gratitude*, the book concludes:

> I cannot pretend I am without fear. But my predominant feeling is one of gratitude. I have loved and been loved; I have been given much and I have given something in return; I have read and travelled and thought and written. I have had an intercourse with the world, the special intercourse of writers and readers.
>
> Above all, I have been a sentient being, a thinking animal, on this beautiful planet, and that in itself has been an enormous privilege and adventure.

Dad, I know, shares Sacks' gratitude. His own special intercourse, with the patients about whom he cared so deeply, means that nothing was ever wasted. Home and work, it all had meaning. He is at peace with his past; indeed, it heightens his present. He is dying with the sense of a life well lived, and I can see how much this helps his departure.

Even as new symptoms reveal themselves, Dad manages to maintain his poise. In this, I suppose, his doctor's training is useful. None of it comes as a surprise to him. He notices odd noises, clicks behind his ears. These are auditory hallucinations, the likely result of his worsening liver failure. He is curious, rather than disturbed by them. Then, the hallucinations escalate. 'Oh fuck,' he suddenly exclaims one morning while brushing his teeth in the bathroom.

Busily counting out his pills, I swivel round in alarm. This is not like my father. 'What is it, Dad? Is it pain?'

'No, it's bloody Tony Blair.'

I raise my eyebrows in bewilderment. At this stage in the game, the last thing I'm expecting is contemporary political history.

Dad elaborates: 'I can see a tiny Tony Blair, right there, sitting on the cold tap, watching me.'

We stare at each other, then burst out laughing.

'Oh Jesus, Dad. I'm so sorry. I mean, dying of cancer is one thing, but *that*? That is just horrible. Horrible.'

He is still muttering 'bloody Tony Blair' and shaking his head in disbelief as I help pull him up to a standing position and we shakily set off along the landing.

'There's something you need to know,' he tells me later. Over the weeks, unbeknown to us all, he has sat down in private and, through the fog of cancer fatigue, written letters to his wife, children and grandchildren. 'They're in a sports bag in my wardrobe, Rachel. You'll find them under my shirts.' This, I realise, is my father's version of Maria's summer fruit and frozen fish. This is love, painstakingly scrawled and sealed inside envelopes, a legacy of words for his family.

Shortly after that, Dad can no longer safely manage the staircase. Each tottering descent fills Mum and me with dread. Nothing could be more awful now than a fall and fractured femur. 'Please, Dad, will you think about a hospital bed?' I plead. He scowls and insists on going outside for a walk, as if to prove how neurotically we are cosseting him. This, most definitely, is madness. It is just before Christmas and bitterly cold, the weather front fresh from Siberia. He has not left the house for a week. He can barely stand, let alone start striding. Yet, refusing assistance, he fumbles defiantly with walking boots, balaclava and Gore-Tex jacket before stomping unsteadily into the frost, armed with his battered trekking poles. I have to grit my teeth and remind myself of my hospice mantra: I help people live what remains of their lives on their own terms, not those of their doctor – or daughter.

My brother and I hastily follow Dad outside, ready to rush to his aid if required. It is cold enough to take our breath away. The wind lashes us viciously. As the fabric of Dad's trousers is whipped against his legs, their outline, essentially, is skeleton. A stooped, cadaverous parody of a fell-walker, he leans doggedly into the gale, his children's hearts splintering behind him. Once he stood with those poles at Everest base camp. Now a handful of yards is all but defying him.

He reaches, at last, the village post box. It is a monumental effort of will that has dragged him here. Behind a wooden bench stands a withered magnolia, gnarled with age and blasted by winter. Every spring, as a child, Dad would show me this tree's annual flowering, an eruption of blooms that delighted him. The magnolia, he would tell me, was one of the most ancient of flowering trees, appearing on Earth some ninety-five million years ago, too soon for the evolution of bees, so relying on beetles for pollination. Once, magnolias had stood alongside Diplodocuses and Tyrannosaurus rexes. I would gaze up at the petals, so white and pure, unable to wrap my mind around numbers this large, concluding, in the end, that the world must have arrived with magnolias fully formed, straight from the primordial swamps of prehistory.

Now, swaying slightly on the grass, Dad inspects the tree carefully. 'It doesn't have long to live,' he pronounces. It is true, I realise, staring at the battered and broken branches. It is dying with Dad, the magnolia of my childhood. He stands before it, frowning silently. I cannot tell if he has drawn a conscious parallel, or if the cold and exertion have stupefied him.

'Shall we go back, Dad?' I ask at last.

The fire is out. He turns, head bowed, and slowly shuffles back towards the family home. My brother, just behind me, is weeping. Watching cancer claim piecemeal a person you love is harder and meaner than I ever knew possible. I think, for the first time, *How long must he endure this?* What I actually mean, though I prefer not to admit this, is: *I can't bear this, it hurts too much, please make it stop now.*

Pain spreads its wings. One day, Dad doubles up in agony under his duvet. We summon the GP, who organises a syringe driver. It works perfectly. Now, no matter how weak or nauseous Dad becomes, a constant trickle of morphine can seep under his skin, keeping the rumbles and flares of pain at bay. He agrees, at this point, to the hospital bed. Holding out against the bed has been his last stubborn stand, his final act of resistance. One tends to assume such a bed belongs upstairs. But Dad does not wish to be banished away like a secret. He wants the bed he knows he will never leave to be placed downstairs, surrounded by the love and life of his family.

Before he begins his last perilous descent downstairs, Mum and I suggest we help him have a shower. The occupational therapy team have provided us with a small seat precisely for this purpose, and I position it just beneath the cascading water. The flow needs adjusting. Dad cannot tolerate a needle-sharp battering. And the temperature too, for those tattered nerve endings. Too cool would be painful; too hot, and his blood would rush to his skin, sending his blood pressure plummeting.

With her nurse's magic, Mum removes her husband's pyjamas and tenderly now, with the utmost care, we ease his gaunt limbs on to the plastic seat, one of us supporting each side of him. Dad sighs, closes his eyes and tilts his face to the water. Slowly, contentedly, he moves his head from side to side, a creature, a mammal, too weary to speak, immersed in its bodily sensations. Droplets catch the light as they bounce from his cheekbones. He opens his mouth to taste the rivulets of water.

'Dad,' I suggest, 'keep your eyes closed. I'll just wash your hair.'

Gently, I lather his scalp with shampoo, soon half drenched myself with foam and water. Then, I turn my attention to this lattice of bones strung together by skin, such a tenuous version of a body. From top to toe, I sponge every inch of my father. These arms that once threw me high above his head, these ribs into which he would enfold his infant children, these shoulders that carried us like proud little monarchs, these thighs I reached towards while learning how to walk. Dad is entirely at ease, his nakedness a state of neither shame nor submission. I have the strongest sense that my mother and I are every bit as exposed as him, flayed by our grief beyond clothes, beyond skin, all the way to our marrow. We could not hide a thing if we tried. And this awkward, cramped, final act of ablution – a husband, a wife and a daughter squeezed into a bathroom built for one – has been transmuted by love into something beautiful. That I can wash my father, as once he washed me, is an honour, an offering, a last act of love, a moment of unrivalled intimacy.

Later that morning, tousle-haired, rosy-cheeked and smelling of Imperial Leather, Dad lays himself down in his hospital bed, especially cushioned to protect his fragile skin. It is almost Christmas and every mantelpiece and window sill is adorned with cards. It is peaceful here, in the corner of the lounge beneath the grandfather clock. He is at the centre of it all, the heart of his home, exactly as he intended.

I leave him sleeping and rush home along the motorway to collect Finn and Abbey. I am worried that the depth of Dad's jaundice and weight loss may frighten them, but I want to give them the chance to say goodbye to their Grampy. Finn, aged eleven, is outraged by the suggestion that he does not need to do so, even if he finds the prospect uncomfortable. 'Of course I want to be there, Mum! I can't even believe you're asking me!' Abbey, at age six, is enthralled by the novelty.

The next day, we spend most of the drive back to Mum and Dad's in intense discussion of cremation versus burial. Abbey, in the end, is seduced by fire. But when she asks if there will be fireworks at Grampy's cremation, I realise her main frame of reference is her recent school bonfire night. She probably has visions of Dad's body bursting into flame on an open-air pyre, like a homemade combustible Guy Fawkes. I am not sure my efforts at preparing the children have been helpful.

When Finn and Abbey arrive at Dad's bedside, they instinctively kiss him and reach out for his hand. There is no horror or apprehension or flinching away. Grampy looks different, but he is still Grampy. Dad watches them both and endeavours to speak. He can only manage the faintest of smiles. Later, at bath time, Abbey is angry. She can see he is too thin and demands to know why we are not giving him food. My explanation that he is too weak to eat cuts no ice with my daughter. She rounds on me and my sub-par doctoring, exclaiming, 'Mummy! You are wrong. He needs an apple a day. Give. Him. An. Apple.'

Day and night, during these final days, Dad's hand is passed from one of ours to another's. Not for one moment is he left alone. What he has given us throughout his life cannot be sold, and what we are trying to give him now is something that cannot be bought.

At night, Mum sleeps by his side on a camp bed, her palm enclosing his until dawn. The syringe driver feeds the drugs that keep his symptoms at bay. He likes the reassuring hubbub of his grandchildren playing nearby. Old enough to understand that Grampy is dying; young enough, seemingly, to take it in their stride, for all his painful emaciation.

You would think Christmas cards and morphine would not mix. But disease does not respect Bank Holidays, and calamity, as we know, can strike at any time. So too can unexpected grace. On Christmas Eve morning, all of us – Dad's three children, three grandchildren and wife of forty-seven years – gather around his bed. It is his birthday. He has turned seventy-five today and, jubilantly led by the children, 'Happy Birthday' makes joy rise from the grief. Though by now he is too weak to smile, his eyes respond with silent delight. He summons all his strength. 'Thank you all,' he murmurs.

By Boxing Day, Dad has reached the hinterland I have been dreading. *Not you, Dad, not you in this life-death limbo I know so well from work.* But here he is, still warm, still breathing – if fitfully now – and yet light years beyond our reach. He lives, but he will never respond to my voice or touch again. I will never know if he hears the words I whisper softly at his side, or feels my hand holding his.

That night, I go to check on Mum, who lies awake on her camp bed, her dying husband's hand in hers, and offer to take her place for a while. But she cannot leave while he lives. This is her gift to my father. Later, in the darkness, I hear her voice at my door. 'Rachel,' she says simply, 'he's gone.'

I am seized by an impulse to scream or howl or beat my chest. I want to tear my hair out. I rush downstairs to my father's bed and clutch him, kiss him, lay my cheek upon his and cling for dear life to the warmth of his limbs, to this last sign of life that, even now, I can feel ebbing away. Desperately, I wrap his hand in mine, cocoon it within my interlocked fingers, as if somehow – if only I can preserve its heat – I will keep him here in the world with me for just a few moments longer.

Like ghosts in the night, the undertakers arrive, solemn and stiff in the frost on the doorstep. It is strange to imagine their emergency summons, as a doctor used to being rushed in the dark to the bedsides only of the living. The men in black suits address the nuts and bolts of mortality – the prompt transportation of the freshly departed – with the utmost tact and civility. Mum closes the door behind them, an ignition key turns, and that is it. All that is left of my father is an imprint of limbs in crumpled bed sheets. We trail uncertainly back to our beds, cut off from each other by the shock of our grief, and curl up in the dark, stunned and reeling.

The next morning, it is hard to believe the sun still shines. I am standing in the kitchen, staring out across fields of frost. Phials of diamorphine are still scattered on the dining room table. The hospital bed needs to go. For a long time, I had not wanted to surface. But, while laid beneath the duvet feeling empty, something unexpected cut through the numbness, my own sudden surge of gratitude. Throughout it all – the major surgery, the countless chemotherapies, the transition from active to palliative care – there were too many acts of tenderness to count. Dad's was a lifetime of service to his NHS patients and, at its end, the NHS could not have repaid him more beautifully.

The technical brilliance of his surgeon, the meticulous skill of the chemotherapy unit, were one thing. But what sung out, over and over, were the innumerable tiny kindnesses which, knitted together, make a patient feel cherished and an NHS hospital so resoundingly humane. There was my father's oncologist, who called him at home on his precious day off with his children. The exhausted nurse on his understaffed ward who took time to hold his hand. The community team who made him feel so special as they tweaked the diamorphine in his final days. None of it would ever count on any official ledger of 'value' – these priceless transactions were not of numbers but of the heart.

On an impulse, still lying in bed, I find myself posting a tweet of thanks to the small army of NHS community nurses who enabled my father to die, as he hoped, at home with his family at Christmas. In Britain, I write, it is easy to forget that when you go through the struggle of a close family death, you are spared the trauma of a large bill at the end of it. We have faced grief, pain and emptiness – but not, at any point, bankruptcy. We have never needed to panic about how we would pay for Dad's care.

Improbably, the tweet sets off around the world, being retweeted some forty-six thousand times and reaching nearly nine million people. The replies, from thousands of men and women I have never met, are overwhelming. An outpouring of kindness and kinship that feels like a living memorial to my newly lost Dad, and to the NHS that cared for him. 'I lost my wife to cancer in October,' writes one man. 'The care and dignity with which she was treated will stay with me for ever.' Another writes: 'I will never forget the debt of gratitude that I felt for the NHS when I was in the same situation and lost my dad.'

Standing at the kitchen sink, I think of the doctor who gave so freely of himself, for so many decades, to his patients. His absence is too large to grasp. Suddenly, a wren darts and whirrs through the hedge in front of me. Dad, in a flash, is there too.

'Look, Rachel! A wren!'

His heart, like mine, never failed to lift at this smallest and most jaunty of birds. The wrens will keep whirring, but he is gone. I walk upstairs to the wardrobe in his bedroom, and rummage in the sports bag for his letters. There they are, seven brown envelopes within which, in virtually indecipherable script, it turns out he still lives after all.

That evening, none of us can face cooking dinner, so I scrape ice off the car and set off for Dad's favourite Indian restaurant to collect us all a curry. The owner, Dad's patient for over thirty years, knows he has been diagnosed with cancer.

'How is your father?' he asks me.

'I'm afraid he passed away last night,' I reply.

'Oh, no, no, I'm so sorry,' he says, and I am startled to see tears welling up in his eyes.

Clutching a bagful of food, I walk out into sub-zero temperatures. The cold bites into my cheeks, but the warmth of his parting words remains: 'Your father, he was such a kind man.'

I do see Dad one more time. On the morning of his funeral, I drive alone to the undertakers where his body is waiting, laid out in its coffin. I presume I will be at home here. I am, after all, an old hand at human corpses. Not a working week goes by without a visit to the mortuary, where my patients lie stacked, sometimes five to a fridge, on gleaming racks that glide on stainless-steel castors. Legally, no patient can meet a crematorium's flames without their doctor first confirming their identity. So, we traipse back and forth, death's stethoscoped secretaries, to sign the forms that enable the release of bodies from the hospital. Cold and bare, too close to abattoir for comfort, I used to recoil at this industrial approach to the logistics of dying. Now, long inured to my inspections of the warehoused dead, I am foolish enough to imagine that seeing my father's body will be easy.

Sure enough, at the funeral parlour, everything is soft and tasteful. Death in disguise, masked by chintz and pastel wall prints. I am shown to the room inside which my father waits and realise I am grateful for the blandness. The last thing I need, with the thump of my heart accosting my ribs, is any hint of starkness. Taking a deep breath, I open the door and enter.

I am on the floor before I realise I have fallen. Felled by the sight of him, my legs cut clean away, crouching now on hands and knees, unable to breathe for sobbing. He has been dressed in the suit he always favoured for weddings, sober and sharp, the colour of charcoal. The tie he is wearing bears the special insignia of a Royal Navy doctor. He planned this all, before he died, every detail of his funeral. Skilled hands have neatly folded Dad's own, one upon the other, and the gaping mouth of his deathbed has been returned to two lips pressed serenely together. His eyelids are closed, his hair neatly combed. I know what tricks of the trade underlie this restoration, but this is entirely irrelevant. You could almost say that this is Dad as he was before cancer. In death, it turns out, there really is resurrection.

All I can think – if you can call this rush of pain thinking – is that the moment I leave this room I will never, ever see my father again. 'Dad,' I cry. 'Daddy.' I cannot stop squeezing his hands and kissing his lips, his cheeks, his brow, his hair, his fingertips. I do not care that he is cold or that his flesh is waxen. I do not give a damn that he lay, wrapped in sheets, inside a fridge this morning. I cannot get close enough to him. I find myself wanting to crawl into the coffin beside him. I even consider it – a moment of madness that is dismissed when I imagine the splintered wood and sheer humiliation of a grown woman breaking into her own father's coffin.

This is it. The final cut, the everlasting severance. I would stay here all day if I could, staving off for as long as possible my last glimpse of my father. Instead, I walk reluctantly out of the door, head twisted backwards towards the open coffin, trying to brand his face on to my retinas.

*

Inside the church, so many family, friends and former patients have assembled that they cannot fit on to the pews. People are standing in the aisles. During the eulogies and hymns, the rituals of departure, I cling to this fact and what it signifies. Afterwards, outside the church, as I am sitting with Mum and my siblings inside the hearse that holds my father, I look out of the window to see Finn, my son, straining his face towards us. He, like his sister, will be cared for by my in-laws while we accompany Dad to the crematorium.

Suddenly, Finn's legs buckle. I see him stagger on the pavement, nearly stumble and fall. His grandmother helps him up, her arms around his shoulders, and as the hearse pulls away, I realise he is sobbing.

Later that night, I ask Finn about what I had witnessed. 'Well,' he tells me, 'I just looked at the coffin inside the car driving off, and I realised I was never going to see Grampy again and it just made me fall over.' There is something uncanny about my son's involuntary response to Dad's death so precisely mimicking mine. I choose to interpret it in terms of a shared depth of love for him, and, a few days later, this seems to be confirmed.

Finn, at the weekend, asks to borrow my laptop. He wants to write about Grampy. It transpires that, at school, his teacher asked for volunteers to speak in assembly about someone they admired. One classmate offered to talk about Nelson Mandela, another to describe Stephen Hawking. Finn, never one to solicit unnecessary homework, immediately asked if he could write about his grandfather.

When Dad, before he died, described how he would outlive his body, I do not think he could have imagined how swiftly and vividly his grandson would bring him to life. Reprinted here, with Finn's permission, are the words he read out to his school, three days after his grandfather's funeral. More than anything, it is the present tense at the start that delights me, the sense of Dad living on:

Grampy

My person that I admire is my Grandpa, but I call him Grampy. I admire him because he always sees the bright side of life; he even thinks clouds are a good thing because of their silver lining. He spreads a sense of positivity wherever he goes.

I also admire him because he always seizes the moment. If he is in Scotland or the Himalayas he will climb mountains. If he is in Greece he would not lie on the beach lazing about, he would spend hours in the sea snorkelling.

He is also very organised (unlike me!). When he was a doctor he created a rota to make sure everyone had the same number of holidays. He would keep the rotas from decades ago to see if someone had missed a day off. He was very determined. If there was a sick patient he would stay there till three in the morning to ensure they were happy. He would even go round to their house and see how they were doing on his day off.

His hobby was to climb mountains. He climbed Mount Kilimanjaro, got to Everest base camp and climbed count-less other mountains. When he was climbing he wasn't only ascending, his spirit was soaring too. This is a picture of him when he had climbed a staggering 5380m to Everest base camp. Sadly he later lost a long and hard battle against cancer and passed away on Boxing Day.

by Finn Clarke

15

Dear Life

*The only calibration that counts is how much heart people invest,
how much they ignore their fears of being hurt or caught out or
humiliated. And the only thing people regret is that they didn't
live boldly enough, that they didn't invest enough heart, didn't
love enough. Nothing else really counts at all.*

Ted Hughes, *Letters of Ted Hughes*

All week the buzz in the hospice has been growing. Everyone
who works here wants the same thing, to give a young bride
a beautiful wedding. The network of caring – so many staff
doing their small part, coming in early, staying late – is spontaneous, impulsive and delightful. Flowers have been ordered,
cupcakes too, and all the staff are bringing in their fairy lights
from home to try and make the day centre look magical. A
volunteer driver will be whisking the groom into town for a
hastily arranged suit-fitting. The white dress should be arriving tomorrow.

Two days is no time at all to organise a wedding. But two

days may be more than we have. Ellie has metastatic breast cancer and she is fading fast. She is so young, only in her early twenties, that for a long time her body resisted her cancer's advances. Now, though, everything is crashing down. Liver failure, kidney failure, a fatigue that creeps into her bones. Daily she grows sleepier and weaker.

As Ellie's doctor, I am torn between recklessness and prudence. She desperately wants to get married on Thursday, with all her friends and family present. Not the wedding of her dreams, of course, but a close approximation, with everyone she loves assembled at her side. Today though, Tuesday, she can scarcely keep her eyes open. I am concerned that at this rate of deterioration, in forty-eight hours she may be unconscious. We could rush a registrar to her bedside at once so that she achieves her ardent wish to marry James, her fiancé. But this would mean forgoing the wedding she has longed for since childhood, an aisle, a cake, a white dress, confetti and – above all – her friends and family sharing the occasion.

'Can you keep me well enough to make it to Thursday?' Ellie asks me. I know such a pledge is not in my gift. All I can do is promise I will try. So I do, as she drifts off to sleep, her skin glowing yellow with jaundice.

Later, I speak separately to James. He understands the risks, he knows the safest course of action. But Ellie has her heart set on a proper wedding. 'Please let's try and give her what she wants,' he tells me.

It is six months since Dad died. After the funeral, I returned to work a different doctor. I have known the taste and weight of grief. Now, when I enter a patient's room, I recognise the sunken eyes and tired frowns of those who cling to the one who would be lost to them. I understand that from the inside out, grief, like love, is non-negotiable, and that the only way to avoid the pain is to opt out of ever loving.

Above all, I have learned from my conversations with my father that being given a terminal diagnosis changes both everything and nothing. Prior to this news, a man of seventy-four, he knew he would die one day, just not when exactly. And after this news, he knew he would die one day, just not when exactly. Everything he had always loved about life was still there to be loved, only more attentively now, more fiercely. All that had changed was the new sense of urgency, the need to savour each day and its sweetness.

'I could waste every day saying, "Why me? Why me?"' Dad once said, 'but I was dying from day one, as we all are. I'll be damned if I let anything but death be the death of me. I'm going to keep on living.'

It rocks me, being back in the hospice. At first, Dad's face confronts me from every pillow. I am back, in a flash, at home beside the hospital bed and the grandfather clock that ticked down Dad's final hours. My patients, however, are still living. And I know that even in the final days there can be moments of staggering sweetness. That in the absence of cure there is still love, joy, togetherness, smiles, tears, wonder, solace – all of life, only concentrated. If anything befits the end of my father's life, it is surely the attempt to ensure that for my patients, these men and women who give us the honour of entrusting their final days to the hospice, dying coexists with living.

Once we know James and Ellie's wishes, we discreetly launch into behind-the-scenes activity. With Ellie too exhausted to focus properly on her wedding herself, she assigns to her three sisters the role of wedding planning. I sit with them late one evening, discovering what we can do to help. Food, decorations, tea cups, cake stands, flowers, music, confetti. So many details that are neither here nor there, or mean absolutely everything, depending on your perspective. As the numbers of invitees grow – first twenty, then forty, then over fifty – we begin to wonder how we will ever squeeze everyone into the day room. 'We'll manage,' says Laurie, the ward sister, firmly. Then she flashes me a smile. 'I admit, it's waking me up at night, but we will manage.'

I grin back. I too am jumping awake in the early hours, but for different reasons. If Ellie drifts into unconsciousness or terminal confusion, she will lose the legal capacity to take part in her wedding. I will have blown her only chance of marrying the man she loves. I know we could rush an emergency registrar to her bedside day or night, but a sudden deterioration could occur at any time – and be fatal. I desperately hope I have not misjudged things.

Thursday morning arrives. I dash to work an hour early. First stop, Ellie's room. There she is, curled up in the arms of her fiancé. They look up sheepishly. Neither James nor Ellie are willing to spend a second apart, regardless of wedding day traditions. 'I don't have time to waste,' says Ellie, smiling at me sleepily. Inwardly, I am cheering. The gamble has been worth it. We will shortly be hosting a wedding.

I gasp as I walk into the day centre. String upon string of white fairy lights already adorn every window and surface. A team of volunteers is working full pelt, racing to make the room perfect. Rows of NHS chairs now define an aisle of sufficient width to permit a wheelchair's entrance. At the front, a plastic table has been disguised with white linen, upon which cream rose petals lie scattered. The bouquets on either side are enormous, luscious. I know the florist we turned to refused point blank to accept any payment. The tower of white-iced cupcakes that form the wedding cake are likewise the gift of a local baker. In an age of atomisation and fractured communities, it turns out that magic string still connects us, after all, human to human – one species.

A little later, I return to check on my patient. The wedding-planning posse has transformed her. Tiny flowers now peep from her hair, her swollen body is hidden beneath folds of white chiffon. She feels no pain, only exhaustion. I leave her to gather her strength for the ceremony.

When Ellie is proudly wheeled by her father down our impromptu aisle, not a person in the room is dry-eyed. You do not need to be a doctor to see how tenuously she clings to life and the world around her. A ghost of a girl, lighter than air, using every last scrap of herself merely to stay in the room with us. There is nothing left with which to smile. I see her head droop for a moment, her eyelids half close. *Come on, Ellie, hold on a little longer.* I hover in a corner, anxiety mounting, ready to intervene if I absolutely have to.

Half-stifled sobs fill the room as the registrar begins the ceremony. But James, I notice, is all smiles. And not just any old smiles. The face-splitting, heart-lifting, cartwheeling kind – foolish and incredulous and bursting with wonder that this woman, this one-in-a-million woman before him, has deigned to be his bride. It is the smile I saw on my own husband's face, all those years ago, the smile I knew I reciprocated.

And, as the ritual continues – those timeworn words of

honouring and committing – I see a change start to creep across Ellie. We are nearing the finale, the moment of marriage, when the strain on her face seems to melt before my eyes. Strangely, slowly, she is being lit from within – first her eyes, then her cheeks, and then, finally, her lips, shyly revealing their own bashful smile. Now it is the room that is shrinking around her. No bashfulness any more, but a kind of exultancy. She grows, glows, and as she says 'I do' she is suddenly, wonderfully luminous. Ellie – no longer a dying young woman, but a bride on her wedding day, radiant, ecstatic. Her cancer vanishes. And everyone sees it, everyone feels it, the world falling away until only one thing remains: two twentysomethings getting married.

The ceremony over, the registry signed, I can see Ellie beginning to list to one side in her wheelchair. She is deflating, collapsing before my eyes.

'Would you like to head back to your room with James?' I whisper.

She nods imperceptibly, too shattered to speak. I explain to the crowd, and the newly weds retreat, waving goodbye to applause that rises and resounds around them like thunder.

Ellie spends twenty-four hours in her husband's arms before drifting into unconsciousness. She dies the next day, still held by James, still wearing her dress of white chiffon.

Sometimes, doctors invent well-meaning stories about dying – that it is entirely painless, effortless, easy. Or, they say something even more outlandish, that death, done 'right', is some kind of transcendent experience, a more lustrous version of ordinary living.

The truth, of course, is that dying is as varied as human experience. There are patterns, for sure, familiar ways in which the body shuts down that we see time and again in the hospice. But a person is irreducible to body parts. Dying can be as banal, harrowing, gentle, brutal, beautiful or frankly prosaic as any other part of human life. For some patients, the predominant sensation is even one of boredom.

In medicine, sugar-coating reality is rarely helpful, however well-intentioned. No matter how skilful the palliative care, there is no softening the enormity of being a living creature who is destined, from the outset, to die. When it comes to matters of life and death, Bob Dylan can usually be relied upon to nail it. 'It frightens me, the awful truth, of how sweet life can be,' he sings in 'Up to Me', a line that I think of, time and again, when pacing the wards of my hospice.

A fusion of awfulness and sweetness: how, in the end, could living be otherwise? For nature is entirely unambiguous in the message she sends us. From the briefest flash of a mayfly in summer to the slow grind of a glacier etching valleys from rock, everything that lives will die, everything is doomed to disappear. No matter how beautiful, no matter how loved, nothing stands still, nothing endures. Impermanence is our only constant.

But against these stark absolutes of lived existence stands something both elastic and enduring: our defining human capacity for *choice*. Our power – one that nothing and no one can take from us – to decide for ourselves how to respond to this fate of being mortal. To rage, to deny, to accept, to embrace. The choice is ours alone.

It takes courage to choose to love the things of this world

when all of them, without fail, are fleeting, fading, no more than a spark against the darkness of deep time. The safest thing, without a doubt, is to shut down, build walls, creep behind barricades – the sensible, sage, irreproachable choice of protecting one's heart, not investing it. Yet Ted Hughes is entirely right. In a hospice, the Death Star, amid the barrage of endings, it is perfectly evident that nothing, in the end, counts but love: how much heart we risk investing in each other. The morphine I prescribe, our clever drugs and infusions, all have undeniable value in keeping pain at bay. But when everything you have been and done and meant to the world is being prised from your grasp, human connections are the vital medicine. It is other people who make the difference.

Perhaps more than any other place on earth, a hospice cleaves apart those aspects of suffering that are necessary – hardwired into the very fact of being human – from the kinds of suffering we can fix or change. Pain, delirium, nausea or fever – such symptoms at the end of life can be tempered immeasurably by medicine's touch, often to a degree that astonishes patients. But the pang and throb of leaving all you hold dear, of being severed from the world you love so ferociously? For this, it is people, not doctors who matter. What I witness, over and over, in the hospice – in this digitised age in which wifi, data and connectivity reign supreme – is that there is nothing more powerful than another human presence, old-fashioned, instinctive, composed of ancient flesh and blood, reaching out with love and tenderness towards one of our own.

If there is a difference between people who know they are dying and the rest of us, it is simply this: that the terminally ill know their time is running out, while we live as though we have all the time in the world. Their urgency propels them to do the things they want to do, reach out to those they love, and savour the moments of life still left to them. In a hospice, therefore, there is more of what matters – more love, more strength, more kindness, more smiles, more dignity, more joy, more tenderness, more grace, more compassion – than you could ever imagine. I work in a world that thrums with life. My patients teach me all I need to know about living.

It is over a year now since my father died. One night, as I am setting off for home from the hospice, I hear music rising from a patient's half-open door. It takes me a moment to recognise those sweeping strings and that crash of brass – the finale of Tchaikovsky's *Swan Lake*. All of a sudden, I see Dad alive again, laughing and applauding from the edge of his seat, as a five-year-old Abbey pirouettes towards him, her eBay tutu twirling furiously, then hurls herself onto the kitchen floor with more panache and commitment than any ballerina in the whole history of dying swans. He hugs her tight as she sits on his knee, bashful at her Grampy's praise, giggling at the scratchiness of his beard.

I smile as I walk away, then find myself drawing to a halt. I know this particular patient has no family or friends. The only company he keeps is the battered radio on his bedside table. Visitors never materialise. I stand still for a moment in the early evening light, hesitating, calculating how much time remains until the children's bedtimes. Then, I retrace my steps towards a dying man's door and, knocking politely, ask if he might let me in.

Postscript

In writing this story, for narrative clarity, I have addressed only briefly several practical matters which a book exploring end of life care cannot, in my view, neglect. I have expanded upon the most important of these here.

Funding

Too many patients, up and down the country, still experience woefully inadequate care at the end of life. Some die in a manner far from their choosing, in great distress and indignity.

This is a national outrage, not to be rose-tinted. If ever an index of humanity mattered, it is surely how generously a society chooses to care for its most vulnerable members, those for whom death is approaching.

Yet extraordinarily, the NHS — supposedly that great bastion of universal care from cradle to grave — funds only a *third* of hospice care in England. The rest — those neglected two-thirds of patients with life-limiting illnesses — are funded by charitable donations: individuals and companies stepping in, in their thousands, where the NHS is failing to deliver. This is a staggering dereliction of care. Imagine the quality of our maternity services or trauma units being contingent on how many jumble sales hit their targets this week. It is almost as though, in times of ever-dwindling government funding, NHS bosses are knowingly exploiting public generosity to quietly short-change the terminally ill.

We could transform the quality of palliative care overnight if it were properly – 100 per cent – funded by the NHS. We could avoid so much unnecessary suffering. A recent ITV News investigation has revealed a UK hospice funding crisis, with increasing demand and rising costs meaning one in three hospices are being forced to cut services, and more than half (55 per cent) having delayed or cancelled their roll out of future plans to increase provision of end-of-life care. Worse, in the past two years, 73 per cent of the hospices have had their local NHS funding frozen or even cut.

This scrimping on hospice funding is occurring at precisely the time when demographic research shows the country's palliative care needs are growing exponentially. As the population both expands and ages, there is likely to be a rise of between 25 and 47 per cent in the number of people needing palliative care by 2040 in England and Wales.

Unless these hard facts are confronted, increasing numbers of people in the UK will die with unnecessary suffering. This is not, primarily, because we cannot face up to death, or because doctors shrink from difficult conversations, but because the resources required to provide high quality, compassionate, patient-centred palliative care for all are simply not there.

In healthcare, amidst the clamour for funds, money tends to follow the loudest voices. Sharp elbows, savvy PR, relentless messaging, celebrity endorsement – these are the ways to win funds for your cause. But the dying speak in whispers, faint and exhausted. Their voices are lighter than air. So it calls upon the living to shout out on their behalf. If we want our loved ones to die with comfort and dignity, we need to lobby MPs, the government and NHS bosses to end this travesty of underfunding.

In a civilised society, palliative care should not be an add-on extra to core NHS services, contingent on whether or not sufficient charitable donations arise. We owe the terminally ill better than that.

Assisted dying

Conspicuous by its absence in this book is a statement of where I stand on the divisive issue of assisted dying.

As the law currently stands, helping someone kill themselves is a criminal offence that carries a maximum sentence of fourteen years. In contrast, providing medical assistance to end a life is legal in various countries such as Holland, Canada, Belgium and Switzerland and in a number of US states.

The UK Parliament last voted on assisted dying in 2015. Then, MPs rejected by 330 to 118 a private member's bill to legalise assistance for those who were terminally ill and likely to die within six months. Yet in opinion polls, around 80 to 90 per cent of the population support this form of assisted dying.

Right-to-die organisations argue that this gulf between politicians and the public shows how out of touch decisions-makers are. The freedom to choose the manner and timing of your own death is, they argue, a fundamental human right. Its denial forces patients to endure unnecessary, avoidable suffering.

In contrast, many judges, parliamentarians, doctors and disability rights groups argue that the law must carefully balance an individual's rights with the need to protect vulnerable people, who may feel pressured, intentionally or unintentionally, into ending their lives. The safest law, they believe, is the one we currently have.

In this book, after much deliberation, I have chosen not to discuss my personal views on assisted dying. For me, the relationship of trust between myself, my patients and their families is paramount, and I worry that expressing my views publicly might jeopardise that bond. A hospice environment is already highly charged with emotion. At work I occasionally encounter patients who are furious with us for not helping them end their lives – yet others are terrified we may secretly use drugs in a syringe driver precisely in order to finish them off. I meet families who argue we would not allow a dog to suffer as their loved one is doing – while the patient, in private, tells us they still want to live. Given the complexity of this real-world context – full of vulnerable patients' hopes and fears – I believe that voicing my personal opinions is at best unhelpful, at worst potentially harmful.

Practical preparations for the end of life

Doctors tend to be obsessed with the importance of planning ahead with respect to death. This is because we so often observe the stress and anguish that can arise from patients, through illness or accident, becoming unable to make decisions for themselves about the care and treatments they would wish for. If, for example, someone suffers a serious brain injury that leaves them in a minimally conscious state, and they have never discussed whether they would wish to be kept alive in such circumstances, their family can feel enormous guilt and anxiety in trying to second-guess what their loved one might wish for.

Advance Care Plans

Advance Care Plans are not legally binding, but they are an important way of ensuring that your family and healthcare professionals know your wishes about care and treatment, if you are no longer able to make decisions for yourself. You can include anything that is important to you such as where you wish to be cared for, who you would want to be with at the end of life, and what your most important values are, such as religious beliefs.

For some people, the prospect of even considering advance care planning, let alone discussing the matter with others, can feel intimidating. A useful downloadable booklet from the organisation www.compassionindying.org.uk, entitled *Starting the Conversation*, aims to support people in talking about their wishes with their family, friends or doctor. It is available here: https://compassionindying.org.uk/wp/wp-content/uploads/2018/04/STARTING-THE-CONVERSATION_2018_AW_SINGLE-PAGES.pdf.

A template plan is available from www.dyingmatters.org. It can be downloaded here: www.dyingmatters.org/sites/default/files/preferred_priorities_for_care.pdf.

Advance Directives

In England and Wales, an **Advance Directive** or **Living Will** is a legally binding means of recording any treatments you do not wish to have in the future, in case you later become unable to make or communicate those decisions yourself. The **Advance Decision to Refuse Treatment**, as it is legally known, will only be used if you cannot make or communicate your decisions yourself. Suppose, for example, you are becoming increasingly frail with metastatic cancer. You might, in those circumstances, decide you do not wish to have cardio-pulmonary resuscitation (CPR) if your heart stops, or to be connected to a ventilator if you cannot breathe on your own. You would record this on the form.

To make an advance directive, you need to complete the form, then sign and date it in the presence of a witness, who also needs to sign and date it. Copies need to be given to your GP and those close to you. A solicitor is not required, so long as you meet the requirements for the form to be legally binding.

A sample form is available here: https://compassionindying.org.uk/library/advance-decision-pack/. Details about how the law differs in Scotland are also available here.

Lasting Power of Attorney

A **Lasting Power of Attorney (LPA)** enables you to give someone you trust the legal power to make decisions on your behalf, in case you later become unable to make decisions for yourself. There are two types of LPA. An LPA for **Property and Financial Affairs** covers decisions about money and property. An LPA for **Health and Welfare** covers decisions about health and personal welfare.

You can complete an official government LPA form online at the government website: https://www.lastingpowerofattorney.service.gov.uk/home. Alternatively, you can download the form here: www.gov.uk/government/publications/make-a-lasting-power-of-attorney. Again, a solicitor is not required for an LPA to be legally valid, provided certain requirements – as detailed on the government website – are met.

Making a Will

A useful guide to **making a will** is available here: https://www.ageuk.org.uk/information-advice/money-legal/legal-issues/making-a-will. A will is a legally binding document ensuring that, when you die, your money and possessions go to the people you would like them to. It is usually safest to use a solicitor to make a will, but you can make your own will. Alternatively, some charities offer free will-drafting services to encourage will making and charitable legacies (although there is no obligation to do so). For example, www.willaid.org.uk provides this service.

More details on all these practical matters can be found on various websites. I find these ones particularly clear and useful:

www.dyingmatters.org
www.compassionindying.org.uk
www.gov.uk/power-of-attorney
www.macmillan.org.uk/information-and-support/organising/planning-for-the-future-with-advanced-cancer
https://deathcafe.com

Credits

Mary Oliver, 'The Summer Day', *House of Light* (Boston, MA: Beacon Press, 1992)

Prologue

Raymond Carver, 'The Author of Her Misfortune', *Ultramarine: Poems* (London: Vintage Books, 1987)

Bob Marley, 'Trenchtown Rock', lyrics © Kobalt Music Publishing Ltd.

Near Misses

Maggie O'Farrell, *I Am, I Am, I Am: Seventeen Brushes With Death* (London: Tinder Press, 2017)

Flesh and Blood

Philip Larkin, 'Ambulances', *The Whitsun Weddings* (London: Faber, 1971)

Skirting Death

Haruki Murakami, *Blind Willow, Sleeping Woman: 24 Stories* (London: Vintage, 2007)

Wit by Margaret Edson, published by and reproduced with permission of Nick Hern Books, www.nickhernbooks.co.uk

Ghost Owl

Susan Sontag, *Illness as Metaphor* (New York: Farrar Straus & Giroux, 1988)

Black Wednesday

Samuel Shem, *The House of God* (London: Black Swan, 1998)

A Numb3rs Game

Stephen Hawking, 'Does God Play Dice?', www.hawking.org.uk/does-god-play-dice.html With the kind permission of United Agents LLP on behalf of the Estate of Stephen Hawking.

Light in the Dark

Sylvia Plath, 'Elm', *Collected Poems* (London: HarperCollins Publishers, 1992)

A Piece of Work

Samuel Beckett, *The Unnamable* (London: Calder Publications, 1975)

Clutching at Straws

Bob Dylan, 'All Along the Watchtower', lyrics © Sony/ATV Music Publishing LLC, Audiam, Inc

Henry Miller, *On Turning Eighty* (Santa Barbara, CA: Capra Press, 1972)

The Price of Love

C. S. Lewis, *A Grief Observed* (London: Faber, 1961)

Wonder

Annie Dillard, *The Writing Life* (London: HarperPerennial, 1990)

Philip Larkin, 'Aubade', *Collected Poems* (New York: Farrar Straus and Giroux, 2001)

Portions of the article 'In Life's Last Moments, Open A Window' by Rachel Clarke originally appeared in the *New York Times* on 8 September 2018

The Man with the Broken Heart

Elastica, 'Connection', lyrics © Warner/Chappell Music, Inc

Gratitude

Henry Miller, *This Is Henry, Henry Miller from Brooklyn* (New York: E. P. Dutton, 1974)

Portions of the article 'Thank you, NHS, for giving Dad the best possible death' by Rachel Clarke originally appeared in *The Sunday Times* on 7 January 2018

Oliver Sacks, *Gratitude* (London: Picador, 2015)

Dear Life

Ted Hughes, *Letters of Ted Hughes* (London: Faber, 2009)

Bob Dylan, 'Up to Me', lyrics © Audiam, Inc, Sony/ATV Music Publishing LLC

Acknowledgements

Heartfelt thanks to my agent Clare Alexander and my editor Richard Beswick for your wisdom, patience, kindness, encouragement and steadfast belief in this book. I could not have been better guided.

Thanks too to Daniel Balado, Zoe Hood, Nithya Rae, Grace Vincent, and everyone at Little, Brown for your support and expertise.

Thank you, Denis Campbell, Kate Fox, Mark Haddon and Rebecca Inglis for reading all or part of *Dear Life*. Your responses were invaluable.

So many conversations with friends have shaped this book. I am hugely grateful to Damian Choma, Moya Dawson, Ed Finch, Alexander Finlayson, Jane Grundy, Jane Henderson, Clare Jacobs, Andy King, Rochelle Lay, Christina Lovell, Robert Macfarlane, Jackie Morris, Natasha Wiggins, Taryn Youngstein – and to Mum, Sarah and Nick.

Tim Littlewood and John Reynolds – you are the doctors I have always looked up to and striven to emulate, alongside my father. Thank you for being such wise, decent and inspiring role models for the next generation.

To all the magnificent NHS nurses I have had the privilege to work with – thank you. You are amazing.

To my patients, who have taught me so much about what matters in life, and for whom it is such an honour to care – my deepest thanks.

And, above all, now and always, all my love and gratitude to Dave, Finn and Abbey.